Praise for

FIT GOD'S WAY

"I've written and co-written several books on diet and exercise, so I'm passionate about these topics. Getting fit and eating 'food' that your body recognizes as food is not easy for anyone, but it's especially tough for women. Women carry the emotional torment of societal pressures to look a certain way and achieve a particular weight or size. The Lord is already using Kim Dolan Leto's Fit God's Way system to heal hearts, create breakthroughs, and form healthy Bible-based habits by putting Him first. This book will transform and possibly revolutionize your relationship with God, yourself, food, and exercise. Highly recommended."

> —**Steve Arterburn,** founder of NewLife Ministries, host of *NewLife Live!* radio, and author of more than one hundred books, including *Every Believer's Thought Life*

"Have you ever asked God to help you become the best version of yourself? Kim's new book *Fit God's Way* is that help! It's like having your own personal health coach cheering you on, page after page, with great spiritual and practical advice that works! I'm so glad Kim wrote this book!"

> —**Wendy Griffith,** CBN news anchor and author of *You Are a Prize to be Won!: Don't Settle for Less than God's Best*

"From the second page in, Kim makes me feel as if I can finally lose the weight I've wanted to lose for the past five years. You know immediately that only the Holy Spirit can help you win the war with yourself to live a life of fitness. I love this book because Kim shows us how this happens. I encourage you to take this journey and become the person God called you to be—mind, body, and soul!"

> —**Cynthia Garrett,** author, TV host, and evangelist

"If you've ever despised exercise or wanted to quit, it's likely because fitness has frustrated you. *Fit God's Way* is God's love letter to you! Women need more than strategies to rev up their metabolism. They want help to activate their faith. Beyond tough coaching, they need relentless grace. Kim encourages women to not just do fitness but to honor God through fitness. *Fit God's Way* strengthens you to fulfill your calling in life—something that Kim has found happens when you know God's love."

—**Brad Bloom,** publisher of *Faith & Fitness Magazine*

"*Fit God's Way* isn't about achieving a look, it's about how you live and who you live for. If you don't know your 'why,' you can't achieve the 'what.' Boldly removing the aesthetic obsession from fitness and finding your spiritual motivation to get fit to serve through your gifts is the turning point of greatness. Kim Dolan Leto has done a masterful job of empowering women to get fit from the inside out, with Christ leading the way."

—**Tana Amen,** vice president of Amen Clinics and *New York Times* bestselling author of *The Omni Diet*

"*Fit God's Way* empowers and teaches us to daily invite God to be part of our fitness journey. By fully relying on the Holy Spirit—our helper—we are never alone, and we have the strength and confidence to see ourselves as God sees us: beautiful and made in His image."

—**Linda Blazy,** CCO of Pure Flix

"Kim Dolan Leto was the faith and fitness expert on *HIS Radio*'s Christian morning show. I'm thrilled to see that same Christ-centered advice packed into one place that everyone can access. Kim is a woman on a mission. She's a powerful voice helping people see the truth: as children of God, we have access to His power, wisdom, and strength, which are the most powerful tools in our health journey."

—**Alison Storm,** host of *HIS Radio* and *My Pleasure: The Unofficial Chick-fil-A Podcast*, and features editor of *Belle Magazine*

Fit God's Way

FIT GOD'S WAY

by Kim Dolan Leto

Follow Kim!

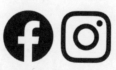

@kimdolanleto

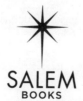

SALEM
BOOKS

an imprint of Regnery Publishing
Washington, D.C.

Scripture quotations marked AMP are taken from the Amplified® Bible, Copyright © 1954, 1958, 1962, 1964, 1965, 1987 by The Lockman Foundation. Used by permission. www.lockman.org

Scriptures marked BSB are taken from the Holy Bible, Berean Study Bible, BSB Copyright ©2016, 2018 by Bible Hub. Used by Permission. All rights reserved worldwide.

Scriptures marked ESV are taken from ESV® Bible (The Holy Bible, English Standard Version®), Copyright © 2001 by Crossway, a publishing ministry of Good News Publishers. Used by permission. All rights reserved.

Scriptures marked ISV are taken from the Holy Bible: International Standard Version® Release 2.0. Copyright © 1996–2012 by the ISV Foundation. Used by permission of Davidson Press, LLC. ALL RIGHTS RESERVED INTERNATIONALLY.

Scripture quotations marked MSG are taken from THE MESSAGE. Copyright © 1993, 1994, 1995, 1996, 2000, 2001, 2002. Used by permission of NavPress Publishing Group."

Scriptures marked NIV are taken from the Holy Bible, New International Version®, NIV®. Copyright © 1973, 1978, 1984, 2011 by Biblica, Inc.® Used by permission of Zondervan. All rights reserved worldwide. www.zondervan.com. The "NIV" and "New International Version" are trademarks registered in the United States Patent and Trademark Office by Biblica, Inc.®

Scripture quotations marked NKJV are taken from the New King James Version.® Copyright © 1982 by Thomas Nelson. Used by permission. All rights reserved.

Scriptures marked NLT are taken from the Holy Bible, New Living Translation. Copyright © 1996, 2004, 2015 by Tyndale House Foundation. Used by permission of Tyndale House Ministries, Carol Stream, Illinois 60188. All rights reserved.

Salem Books™ is a trademark of Salem Communications Holding Corporation.

Regnery® and its colophon is a registered trademark of Salem Communications Holding Corporation.

ISBN: 978-1-68451-264-5
eISBN: 978-1-678451-320-8

Cover Photograph by The Ivory Curator

Published in the United States by

Salem Books
An Imprint of Regnery Publishing
A Division of Salem Media Group
Washington, D.C.
www.SalemBooks.com

Manufactured in the United States of America

10 9 8 7 6 5 4 3 2 1

Books are available in quantity for promotional or premium use. For information on discounts and terms, please visit our website: www.SalemBooks.com.

For from Him and through Him and to Him are all things.

To Him be the glory forever! Amen.

CONTENTS

Habit 4:
Choose Fit Thoughts

Habit 5:
Eat to Fuel Your Temple

Habit 6:
Make Fitness Holy

Habit 7:
Press On—Don't Quit!

Introduction

The Promise

My promise to you . . .

What would it take for you to let me help you live free from the dieting cycle of losing and gaining weight and the emotional torment it causes? How would you feel if this whole weight and body image struggle were gone? What if you knew what to eat, had motivation to work out, and felt good in your body? What if I gave you a plan based in the Word and promised to be your "Fit-Sister-in-Christ Success Coach," equipping you with the blueprint from the beginning to the end?

Would you join me?

I've personally gone through this battle and taken thousands of women through it with this Bible-based answer that works. Twenty years ago, God pulled me out of a pit of hopelessness and transformed my tired, overweight, and out-of-shape body and life into one on a mission to teach Christ as the centerpiece of fitness.

Chances are, you've tried a lot of diets, but the results didn't last. You've joined a gym and maybe even bought home equipment, but your motivation faded. You've broken self-made promises to eat better, you've skipped workouts, and your confidence and body image have suffered in the process.

I know the desperation to want to lose weight. I've lived it. I tried doing what the world offered, but my motivation never lasted. I stood on the scale and looked in the mirror and felt the shock of *How did I get here?*

You too?

Friend, don't be hard on yourself. You're not alone in this struggle. Jesus not only cares about every detail of your fitness and wholeness, He gave you a helper—the Holy Spirit—to guide you, comfort you, and strengthen you.

Here is my promise to you, if you read this book and apply these truths to your life:

1. The cycle of losing and gaining weight and the emotional chaos it causes will cease, and you will have peace.
2. You will have a doable and sustainable plan that works in your life and is built on the Word.
3. You will know God's love for you and His promise to lead, guide, strengthen, and pick you back up in His grace.

I wrote *Fit God's Way* for women like you and me who hurt deeply over our battle to be fit. We've struggled alone in silence, and we've spent way too much time thinking about the way we look and feeling defeated. We've suffered alone, and we need a friend to show us the way. Let me be that friend.

There are seven habits in *Fit God's Way*. They were created from coaching women and seeing what they needed to find a lasting answer to their fitness. These habits put God first in your fitness, and they are your proven foundation. Within each of the habits, you will hear stories from other women and get the same Bible-based solutions, scriptures, prayers, action steps, charts, and tips that ended their struggles and led them to success.

I made the number seven a focus of this book because of the Biblical significance behind it. Seven is the number of completeness and perfection (both physical and spiritual).[1] While there is no perfection this side of Heaven, our Jesus is perfect—and in Him, we can experience completeness and become the very best versions of ourselves.

The 7 Habits of *Fit God's Way*

Habit 1: Put God First in Your Fitness
Learn to end the cycle of dieting failures and put God first in your fitness.

Habit 2: Get Fit God's Way with the 7 Ws
Get the framework for your personalized daily system, set goals, and take part in the #FitGodsWay Challenge.

Habit 3: Activate Your Faith
Learn the importance of believing God before seeing results, and get helpful tools to start taking action.

Habit 4: Choose Fit Thoughts
Find worth, identity, and power by seeing His perfection in your reflection.

Habit 5: Eat to Fuel Your Temple
Get a mini-course in weight loss and nutrition basics, and learn how to eat God-made foods, how to make a God-made plate, and tips for grocery shopping, prep, and cooking.

Habit 6: Make Fitness Holy
Gain a heart of wisdom to motivate your workouts, and make them an act of worship to get fit from the inside out.

Habit 7: Press On—Don't Quit!
Learn to honor God in your body beyond fitness, and get tools to help you overcome what makes you want to give up.

If you're a Christian woman who loves Jesus and fitness, the seven Fit God's Way Habits will provide Bible-based answers for every aspect of your fitness and body image and will enable you to create a Spirit-led, fit lifestyle.

If you're tired of starting your diet over every Monday, if getting dressed stresses you out, or if scrolling through your social media feed makes you feel insecure, *this is not of God!*

The way the world portrays health, fitness, and body confidence causes us to live in a thought cycle of feeling defeated and "not good enough," but in Christ, we are free to live boldly as the best version of ourselves. This book is not about perfection or being enslaved by body-part idolatry, but rather, freedom, wholeness, and power through Christ.

You can cross the finish line of your goals. You just need to build your Fit God's Way system.

I believe God led you to this book for a reason. Maybe fitness has been a deep place of struggle for you, maybe you're tired of looking in the mirror and not seeing the fearfully and wonderfully made woman of God you are, or maybe you want to experience Him in a whole new way in your fitness and wholeness. My prayer is that you find exactly what you need to become the very best version of yourself for Him. You are a daughter of the King, you have access to power, wisdom, and strength, and now is your time. You have been called, set apart, and chosen for such a time as this.

Are you in? All you have to do is keeping turning the pages.

> Now all glory to God, who is able, through his mighty power at work within us, to accomplish infinitely more than we might ask or think. (Ephesians 3:20 NLT)

Fit God's Way Challenge

Hey there, Fit Sister-in-Christ.

I have a feeling you want to start making changes right away, and I bet you want a plan to follow to jumpstart your results. Well, I've got you covered. I'd like to invite you to take the #FitGodsWay 7 Ws Social Media Challenge.

Here's how: Post a picture of you doing one or all of the 7 Ws with #FitGodsWay on social media. If you're wondering how to get started, here are some simple ideas to help:

- Take a picture of yourself praying or reading your Bible, sharing how you find worth in Christ through favorite Scriptures, quotes, and even how you give yourself grace when you miss a goal.
- Share images of yourself eating God-made food and drinking water out of your go-to container.

- Snap a photo of yourself working out, listening to your favorite worship song, and share how you do your morning and evening routine.

Love freebies? Want more tips? Download your free Fit God's Way 7 Ws checklist, and find workouts, recipes, and motivation at www.fitgodsway.com.

Fit God's Way Daily 7 Ws

Word: Read your Bible and pray.

Worth: Practice placing your worth in Christ to find confidence, strength, and grace.

Whole, God-Made Food: Choose whole, God-made food over processed, man-made foods. Focus on quality ingredients versus obsessing over quantities. Pray before meals.

Water: Divide your weight in half and drink a minimum of that many ounces per day. Add seven to ten ounces of fluid every ten to twenty minutes during exercise.

Work Out: Move and strengthen your body five to six days a week. In addition, take walks outdoors to spend time in God's creation and mini-movement breaks throughout the day to increase your non-exercise activity calorie burn.

Worship: Listen to Christian music, sing, dance, and praise God.

Wake/Sleep: Establish a wake/sleep cycle and a morning/evening routine to put yourself to bed in the peace of God and wake up in His power.

Within these pages, you will learn everything you need to know about the 7 Ws. But for now, I challenge you to jump in and start getting fit God's way.

I'll be cheering you on and praying for you,

Kim Dolan Leto

HABIT 1:

Put God First in Your Fitness

How to Put God First in Your Fitness

Trust in the Lord with all your heart,
And lean not on your own understanding;
In all your ways acknowledge Him,
And He shall direct your paths. Do not be wise in your own eyes;
Fear the Lord and depart from evil. It will be health to your flesh,
And strength to your bones.

Proverbs 3:5–8 NKJV

Has this ever happened to you? You walk into your closet to get dressed, and as you try on outfits, a conversation starts in your mind—thoughts like, *I need to lose weight, I need to start working out more, I hope no one notices the weight I've gained.* You find nothing seems to fit right, and it's making you miserable. You frantically change a few times before finally settling on your go-to outfit for *those days.*

How many times have you promised to eat cleaner, to work out, to try harder next time? But then no matter how hard you try, you always seem to give up. Life gets busy, the kids get sick, or the results don't come fast enough. There just doesn't seem to be enough motivation to keep you focused, but deep down, you know there's a better version of you. You long to be her, to be free of all this, but you push these thoughts of a better you aside for when you have more time.

Somewhere between criticizing your body and promising to do better, you never made this connection. Instead, you fight this battle on your own, and you live in a prison of wrong thoughts. Struggling with your body image and trying to get fit and feel comfortable in your skin seem like things you could never ask God about, or even consider praying for, so you suffer in silence, feeling less-than.

In your heart you love God, and you love fitness. But maybe no one ever told you that they need to be done together to work correctly?

End the Cycle of Dieting Failure by Seeking God First in Your Fitness

Have you ever wondered:

- If God cares about your struggles with food and fitness?
- How to get your eating under control?
- Why it's so hard to stay motivated?
- How to have a healthy body image?
- Why worldly fitness answers don't work?

As our answer to fitness unfolds in these pages, we will see how Jesus cares about every detail of our lives—yes, even our fitness struggles. We'll also learn that He gave us a helper, the Holy Spirit, why His plans for us are our greatest motivation, that we are fearfully and wonderfully made, and that the answers to our fitness issues are only found in Him.

Jesus is our perfect role model because:

- He rose early.
- He spent time with His Father.
- He prayed about everything.
- He wasn't lazy.

- He enjoyed food.
- He ate to live; He didn't live to eat.
- He walked everywhere.
- He loved people.
- He came to serve.
- He wasn't concerned with what others thought about Him.
- He lived for God and to fulfill the plan for His life.
- And He finished His race with endurance!

The habit of putting God first in our fitness is based on following Jesus's example and knowing that He gave us a helper, comforter, and counselor to live this fit life—the Holy Spirit.

> "But the Helper, the Holy Spirit, whom the Father will send in My name, He will teach you all things, and bring to your remembrance all things that I said to you." (John 14:26 NKJV)

For those of us who follow Jesus, the reason fitness hasn't worked in the past is that we've left Him out of it. Think about it: How many times have you gone to church on Sunday and then out to eat with your family? When Monday came, you promised to start eating better then turned to the world for your fitness answers. For those of us who love Jesus, seeking answers apart from Him won't work. God must be first in everything in our lives—every aspect. Wherever He's not will be a place of pain, confusion, and struggle.

Seeking God first gives Him His rightful place and teaches us a completely new perspective on taking care of ourselves.

> "But seek first the kingdom of God and His righteousness, and all these things shall be added to you." (Matthew 6:33 NKJV)

Now, I'm not saying that if you seek God first in your fitness that all of a sudden, the weight will just fall off and your confidence will skyrocket.

God is not some genie in a bottle or the new secret to fat loss. What I am saying is that if you put Him first and acknowledge Him in all your ways, He will give you wisdom and guide you to the right path to health.

"We cannot give our hearts to God and keep our bodies to ourselves."
—Elisabeth Elliot

Sometimes our limited understanding of God and our intense desire to reach a goal is the very thing keeping us from it. God wants all of us—our mind, body, and soul—living for Him. In doing so, we find the life He died to give us.

> Then He said to them all, "If anyone desires to come after Me, let him deny himself, and take up his cross daily, and follow Me. For whoever desires to save his life will lose it, but whoever loses his life for My sake will save it." (Luke 9:23–24 NKJV)

Giving God all of us and denying ourselves removes the flesh-driven spirit from fitness and replaces it with a Spirit-led lifestyle. As Christians, we often follow people who aren't following God, and when we do, their influence pollutes and distracts us from God's plans for our lives. Truly, we shouldn't be following anything or anyone who isn't following Jesus, because their ways are not our ways. The success we're looking for in our health and wholeness doesn't come from others or ourselves; it comes from putting God first.

How to Make Putting God First in Your Fitness a Habit

This is how we put God first in our fitness: We seek Him. We spend time with Him and in His Word. We pray about everything. We choose not to be lazy or gluttonous. We eat the foods He made for us. We move our bodies. We choose to serve people through our gifts. We don't concern ourselves with what others think of us. We live to fulfill His plan for us. We run our race with endurance.

We were made by God for God. We are not here for ourselves.

Why the Habit of Putting God First in Your Fitness Works

- God said if we acknowledge Him in all our ways, He will direct our paths.
- We have a helper, the Holy Spirit.
- We can have peace with ourselves now, not just when we reach a goal.
- Our worth is hidden in Christ and no longer tied to numbers.
- We have power in His promises.
- We can stop the cycle of undereating, overeating, stress eating, and bingeing because we go to God with our emotions. We learn to stop eating our emotions or numbing ourselves with food to cope with our problems.
- Through Him, we can repair and find a healthy relationship with food.
- We are set free from valuing ourselves based on performance, so we don't have to feel like failures.
- We can stop obsessing over the way our bodies look and actually take care of ourselves.
- We don't think about food all the time.
- We stop believing the world has some magic answer to help us lose weight or get fit.
- We stop looking for quick-fix answers in pills, powders, and packaged food.
- We eat what God made for us with prayer and thanksgiving.
- We're free in Christ to enjoy food without guilt and feel good in our skin.
- When we fall off track, we run to the Word, and God picks us up in His grace.
- We invest in ourselves in order to do the work through a Spirit-led lifestyle for Kingdom purposes.

As we learn the habit of putting God first in our fitness, we find freedom from worldly standards and dieting schemes, and we find satisfaction in how He formed us—uniquely and without mistake.

We enjoy the foods He made for our bodies with prayer and thanksgiving and without obsessive dieting, overeating, or undereating, which leads to emotional torment. We train our bodies toward health to fulfill the call He has on our lives rather than achieving an aesthetic ideal. And while our fit bodies and healthier lifestyles are side effects of this newly found lifestyle, His plans and purposes for us are where we thrive and find our lasting motivation and significance.

> **"I will instruct you and teach you in the way you should go; I will counsel you with my loving eye on you."**
> —Psalm 32:8 NIV

You Are Not Alone in Your Fitness

The habit of putting God first in our fitness is the answer our hearts have been looking for, because only God can meet each of us individually in our stories and give us the answers we need and the daily grace to keep going. In Him, we have power and access to the wisdom, strength, confidence, peace, and endurance to live fit lifestyles.

Let us therefore come boldly to the throne of grace, that we may obtain mercy and find grace to help in time of need. (Hebrews 4:16 NKJV)

Chapter 1

Redefining Fitness God's Way

The Bible has the answer to every question, the solution to every problem. It is our instruction manual for life, including our fitness!

I had a come-to-Jesus moment with my health in 1999 that changed me forever: I learned my father had just had a stroke. I can still remember the bright hospital lights and the lack of sleep I felt that day. The combination made me hope I was dreaming and that when I woke up, it wouldn't be true. I could hear a doctor saying words like, "paralysis, stroke, and quadruple bypass," and the shock of them was gripping. I ran to the bathroom and prayed through tears that God would heal my father, but things didn't look good.

As I left the hospital in a haze, I could hear God saying, "You need to take your health seriously." I had just gotten blood work done, and it showed that my cholesterol was high. Between that and being thirty pounds overweight, I could feel panic coursing through my veins. I was scared, but I didn't know how to start getting fit.

This was over twenty years ago, so all the fitness resources we currently have weren't available. The first thing I did was call my church. I asked them to pray for my dad and whether they had any fitness groups or health advice, but they didn't. So I drove to a bookstore and bought a bunch of fitness books and magazines. Once I was home, I combed over every word, every picture, and every workout move, taking exhaustive notes.

All the while, I couldn't get the picture of my father lying in the hospital bed out of my mind. My heart ached for him. I felt ashamed that I had allowed myself to get so unhealthy. I never exercised, and I ate poorly. I was overweight and out of shape. I had never made fitness or healthy eating a part of my life. But now, I was desperate to get fit.

I Did Fitness the Wrong Way

My dad ended up having quadruple bypass surgery. The stroke left him with paralysis in his face and the entire left side of his body. The scar on his chest and the way the paralysis affected his face were a constant and painful reminder of all he went through—and that motivated me in fearful way. Looking back, I wish I had known that I could go to God. I was never taught to go to Him or that it's okay to pray for His help with getting healthy. So I did what I think most of us do in those situations: I went to the world.

The fitness magazines and books made something come alive in my flesh. In a magazine called *Oxygen*, I remember seeing pictures from an ESPN Fitness America competition. Years before, when I was in college, I had watched that competition and for absolutely no reason grounded in reality, I thought, *I'm going to compete in that one day.*

I knew I needed a big goal to get fit, so I made the Fitness America competition my time-based goal. I found an event eleven weeks out and nervously signed up.

Now, I have to be real with you: this was beyond far-fetched! My friends and family all but laughed at me. They said things like, "Yeah, right! And you're going to do what?!" Even my husband asked, "So you know how to do gymnastics?" I said, "No, but I can learn."

Picture it: I was barely able to do a pushup, and I had a lot of weight to lose. But I knew I needed to make extreme changes. I called around and found a gymnastics center that had adult classes; I started going three days a week and putting a routine together. I had never taken dance lessons, so I watched what the top fitness competitors did and tried my best to choreograph a routine. I'm Latin, so my first theme was a Latin one. (It's embarrassing to think about this, because I really didn't know what I was doing.) I tore out the pages of workouts from my fitness magazines, began training five days a week, and eating like the magazines said to. I was working full-time, so this life change took everything out of me. I was constantly sore, everywhere.

My body started to change very slowly. The scale didn't move much the first month because I was gaining lean mass and my bodyfat was decreasing. At around week six, there was a visible difference in my midsection. The combination of removing unhealthy, processed foods from my diet, overly restricting my calories, and consistently exercising was transforming my body. The day before my competition, I took my measurements and couldn't believe I had lost eight inches off my waist.

> "For it is God who works in you both to will and to do for His good pleasure."
> —Philippians 2:13 NKJV

After eleven weeks of training and dieting, my family and I flew to Montana for my first competition. My dad came, and he was so proud of me. My family and friends said they didn't even recognize me. At the show, I was so nervous. I had no idea what I was doing, but I ended up placing third.

Fitness Is a Battle between Flesh and Spirit

When I got home from the competition, I started feeling the extremes of fitness. Within just a few days of eating normally, my body looked heavier and less defined, and my original passion to be healthy now felt more like a pick-myself-apart perfection project. The competition in Montana landed me an invitation to compete at the Fitness America Nationals, so I felt pressure to be leaner, and the numbers on the scale and between the calipers started to become an idol.

Throughout my competition days, in my morning time with God, He started speaking to my heart. I remember writing in my journal, "Where is God in any of this?" I didn't like how this part of my life felt so separate from Him. I started getting really convicted and confessed to Him that I had made fitness an idol. I asked Him to forgive me and to help me, and He led me to Scripture and gave me real answers that worked.

These are the tools you will learn throughout this book that have helped countless women break free from the grip of flesh in fitness.

I have to share that at one of my competitions, I met the editor of *Oxygen*, the very magazine that initially helped me start getting fit, and she asked me to be on the cover. When the staff asked, "What's your secret to staying fit?" I shared how I prayed before meals, ate God-made foods, and how I wanted to be fit for the purposes and plans God had for me. Of course, the magazine never published any of that. I was surprised they still put me on the cover. I was thirty-six years old at the time. (I think God must have a sense of humor, because I was forty-eight years old on my last cover.)

After my final fitness competition in 2011, my family and I decided to celebrate by going to a beautiful lake where I live in Arizona. As I was walking behind my husband and our sweet little girl, I heard these words: "*F.I.T.: Faith Inspired Transformation. Tell people the truth about your fitness experience and what really works.*" In that moment, I knew I needed to share how I was able to get fit and finally feel at peace within my body.

When I look back, I clearly see how God allowed me to do fitness in the flesh, because it was my life's purpose to share how unhealthy fitness is without Him—but that in Him is every answer we need.

Fitness without God Is a Frustrating Flesh Project

During the times I felt disappointment from not being able to keep my weight down, eat perfectly, or look perfect, God showed me that fitness without Him is a flesh project. This is why it doesn't work. There is a constant war within a believer between the Spirit and the flesh. What I have experienced while working with thousands of women and myself is that when fitness is all about what you look like, you're never satisfied. Our flesh is always searching for the easy way and for more and, in the process, it makes you feel like less. The flesh picks you apart and points out every flaw. *If only my thighs were smaller or my waist were narrower.* This dissatisfaction and division within ourselves is not of God. The flesh is incapable of being satisfied.

The Bible tells us:

"If a house is divided against itself, that house cannot stand." (Mark 3:25 ISV)

For where envy and self-seeking exist, confusion and every evil thing are there. (James 3:16 NKJV)

Those who live according to the flesh have their minds set on what the flesh desires; but those who live in accordance with the Spirit have their minds set on what the Spirit desires. The mind governed by the flesh is death, but the mind governed by the Spirit is life and peace. The mind governed by the flesh is hostile to God; it does not submit to God's law, nor can it do so. Those who are in the realm of the flesh cannot please God. (Romans 8:5–8 NIV)

I say then: Walk in the Spirit, and you shall not fulfill the lust of the flesh. For the flesh lusts against the Spirit, and the Spirit against the flesh; and these are contrary to one another, so that you do not do the things that you wish. (Galatians 5:16–17 NKJV)

Meet Sarah

Sarah wanted help losing the weight she had gained during the pandemic. She almost cried when she said none of her clothes fit anymore and she now had to go back into the office for work. She had tried just about every diet and was desperate. Sarah said, "I do really well for the first few days, sometimes even a couple weeks, but I obsessively weigh myself to the point that all I can think of is that number, and I'm so tempted by food, I feel like I'm at war with myself."

When I told Sarah that she wasn't alone—that even Jesus was tempted with food—she was shocked. We read this scripture together:

> Then Jesus was led up by the Spirit into the wilderness to be tempted by the devil. And when He had fasted forty days and forty nights, afterward He was hungry. Now when the tempter came to Him, he said, "If You are the Son of God, command that these stones become bread." But He answered and said, "It is written, 'Man shall not live by bread alone, but by every word that proceeds from the mouth of God.'" (Matthew 4:1–4 NKJV)

It may feel like Jesus couldn't possibly relate to your struggles, but the Bible says, "For we do not have a high priest who is unable to empathize with our weaknesses, but we have one who has been tempted in every way, just as we are—yet he did not sin." (Hebrews 4:15 NIV) Jesus was tempted just as we are, so He knows exactly what we're going through and how to help us overcome it. It may surprise you to know that your temptations are no surprise to God, but in Him, you can escape them. We face spiritual battles and strongholds when it comes to food, fitness, and our body image, and the problem is that we try to solve them with answers apart from God. Maybe, like Sarah, you have thought *Why can't I stick to my diet?* But it isn't the food or the workouts that are your problem—it's much deeper than that. Think of the diets you've tried in the past. Were their results long-lasting? Did any of it make you feel healthier, happier, or closer to the godly woman you want to be?

Why Diet Results Don't Last

The enemy preys on our insecurities and weaknesses and wants to steal our health.

"The thief comes only to steal, and to kill and to destroy. I have come that they may have life, and that they may have it more abundantly." (John 10:10 NKJV)

I once heard someone say the devil doesn't come with a pitchfork and horns looking evil. He comes dressed up like everything you've ever wanted. You may be wondering what this has to do with your fitness; the answer is, the enemy knows this is a place of struggle for you.

The devil has a foothold in the fitness industry. He's made it a flesh project—not a health or wholeness project. He torments us about our fitness by tempting us into cycles of unhealthy behavior, overeating, overtraining, undereating, not exercising at all—and then shames us. There's a constant war for our mind, and he knows exactly how to keep us stuck in a cycle of failure.

This is why we are told in Ephesians 6:10–14 to put on the armor of God.

Finally, my brethren, be strong in the Lord and in the power of His might. Put on the whole armor of God, that you may be able to stand against the wiles of the devil. For we do not wrestle against flesh and blood, but against principalities, against powers, against the rulers of the darkness of this age, against spiritual hosts of wickedness in the heavenly places. Therefore take up the whole armor of God, that you may be able to withstand in the evil day, and having done all, to stand. (NKJV)

Think of the last time you tried to get fit. Does any of this ring true?

The enemy lures you in with how you're going to look, lies to you, and leaves you feeling less-than. He gets you so busy and preoccupied with your weight and your body that you begin living in your head, consumed with how you look and what others think of you.

Once you're trapped in this cycle, fitness has become an idol, and you're on a rollercoaster of falling for get-fit-quick promises and perhaps the approval of others.

You may even exhaust yourself with perfectly posed and filtered selfies to show your fit body—but the subsequent emptiness and dissatisfaction within leaves you with a gaping hole in your heart and paralyzing insecurity. Can you see the sway of the wicked one here?

> We know that we are of God, and the whole world lies under the sway of the wicked one. And we know that the Son of God has come and has given us an understanding, that we may know Him who is true; and we are in Him who is true, in His Son Jesus Christ. This is the true God and eternal life. Little children, keep yourselves from idols. Amen. (1 John 5:19–20 NKJV)

Flesh-driven fitness is a trap for three main reasons:

1. It's an idol. It never produces lasting results for those of us who love Jesus, because He must be first in all things. Anything we put before Him is an idol, and God will have no gods before Him.
2. It creates an unhealthy, warped relationship with food and your body. You feel great when you eat right and like a failure when you don't. This relationship is shame- and performance-based and ungodly. You weren't created to think about what you eat and how you look all the time.

3. It doesn't have a power source. In the flesh, you're on your own. You don't have God or the Holy Spirit.

Dieting and Body-Image Statistics

These statistics clearly illustrate that we need a deeper answer for our health problems:

- Seventy-two billion dollars a year is spent on diet aids.[1]
- Seventy-four percent of adults are overweight or obese.[2]
- Eighty to 95 percent of people gain back all the weight they lose on diets.[3]
- Obesity rates are higher for women.[4]
- Thirty-five percent of "occasional dieters" progress into pathological dieting (disordered eating), and as many as 25 percent turn into full-blown eating disorders.[5]
- According to U.S. News & World Report, a whopping 80 percent of New Year's resolutions fail by February.[6]
- Eighty-nine percent of American women are unhappy with their weight, and 84 percent would like to lose weight.[7]

Trade Fitness in the Flesh for Fitness in the Spirit

Have you ever considered the team of highly trained marketing, advertising, communications, and social media specialists, as well as all the stylists, makeup artists, photographers, and editing software involved in dieting and fitness advertising?

Picture the side-by-side before-and-after images of perfect body parts used to sell fitness products. These images are intentionally curated to feed our flesh. They make us believe that we don't have to actually work for our results, because the product being sold is the quick way to get the weight off and look great. What they're selling us is a feeling, hope for a better version of ourselves, and a lie that there's a fast way to get there with minimal work on our part. What does the Word say about this? Beware, and be wise!

> Beware lest anyone cheat you through philosophy and empty deceit, according to the tradition of men, according to the basic principles of the world, and not according to Christ. (Colossians 2:8 NKJV)

> "Behold, I send you out as sheep in the midst of wolves. Therefore, be wise as serpents and harmless as doves." (Matthew 10:16 NKJV)

We've all fallen for a good marketing scheme before, and that's okay, but we shouldn't continue falling for the deception. Brian Hardin, the creator and voice of the Daily Audio Bible, once said something that sums up this type of fitness experience perfectly: "What we really need is God, not whatever quick fix we're looking for."

We've been taught from a young age that dieting is how we lose weight, and we've relied on worldly answers because we've also been taught that fitness is pursued separately from God—but it shouldn't be.

> Therefore, whether you eat or drink, or whatever you do, do all to the glory of God. (1 Corinthians 10:31 NIV)

Maybe you've tried a lot of diets, but you haven't found lasting results. You feel hopeless and long to feel good in your skin again. Search your heart and ask yourself if you've been trying to get healthy without God. Where does He fit into your fitness? Has fitness become an idol? What about the scale, certain body parts, social media, or the approval of others? These all indicate you are pursuing fitness in the flesh.

God's Spirit Conquers Our Flesh

"And I will give you a new heart, and a new spirit I will put within you. And I will remove the heart of stone from your flesh and give you a heart of flesh. And I will put my Spirit within you, and cause you to walk in my statutes and be careful to obey my rules." (Ezekiel 36:26–27 ESV)

As a believer in Jesus Christ, you have the Holy Spirit living in you. You no longer have to do fitness alone and in your own abilities. You don't have to listen to that inner critic that points out every poor food choice or every skipped workout, and you can learn to like yourself the way God made you and your body. When you make the decision to get fit God's way, you have promises that result in power and peace.

God Provides the How-To and the Want-To

Growing in God is the goal of Fit God's Way. So if you're Christian, but you're not really sure about how you get this power and peace—the Holy Spirit—I want to share some helpful basics to make you aware of the gift God has given you.

- When you became a Christian, God sent His Spirit to live in you.
- God knew we would need help living this Christian life, so He sent us the Holy Spirit to empower and guide us. Acts 1:8 tells us that Jesus said, "But you shall receive power when the Holy Spirit has come upon you; and you shall be witnesses to Me in Jerusalem, and in all Judea and Samaria, and to the end of the earth." (NKJV)
- Each of us has gifts from the Holy Spirit. First Corinthians 12:8–10 (NIV) lists the following: "To one there is given through the Spirit a message of wisdom, to another a message of knowledge by means of the same Spirit, to another faith by the same Spirit, to another gifts of healing by that one Spirit, to another miraculous powers, to another prophecy, to another distinguishing between spirits, to another speaking

in different kinds of tongues, and to still another the interpretation of tongues." If you have no idea what your gift is, find a spiritual gifts test online to discover yours.

- The fruits of the Spirit are how you can see God working in you. Think of God as the root or the vine and our actions (because of His character growing in us) as the fruit. When you hear the term "fruit," think of an action and a result to gain a clearer understanding of what it means to have the fruit of the Spirit. Ask yourself if you see these fruits, and thank God for working in you to bring them out for His glory. "But the fruit of the Spirit is love, joy, peace, patience, kindness, goodness, faithfulness, gentleness, self-control; against such things, there is no law." (Galatians 5:22–23 ESV)
- The Holy Spirit is there to lead you daily to a new life in Christ.
- When you don't know what to do, you can ask the Holy Spirit to guide you.
- The Holy Spirit will bring scriptures to mind when you need them.
- The Holy Spirit will make you aware of things that are not of God or His will.
- The Holy Spirit is your comforter, counselor, healer, guide, and strength. He equips you to be bold to live for God.

The Holy Spirit is often referred to as a *still small voice*, but He is so much bigger than that. God loves us so much that He sent His Son, Jesus, to die for our sins. Before Jesus died and rose again, He promised to send us a Helper.

For God so loved the world that He gave His only begotten Son, that whoever believes in Him should not perish but have everlasting life. For God did not send His Son into the world to condemn the world, but that the world through Him might be saved. (John 3:16–17 NKJV)

"Nevertheless, I tell you the truth. It is to your advantage that I go away; for if I do not go away, the Helper will not come to you; but if I depart, I will send Him to you." (John 16:7 NKJV)

Take a deep breath, close your eyes, and picture yourself reaching out to God. Envision His hand guiding you on your new journey to health and wholeness in Him. He loves you, and He cares. He wants you to go to Him with your dieting struggles, help you find the right workout, and overcome body-images issues. Trust in Him; place each day, your goals, and your gifts in His hands. Begin taking the very best care of yourself to bring Him glory and become the godly woman you really want to be. The companionship of God's indwelling Holy Spirit and His Word are the best fitness coaches, because His unconditional love and grace upholds us, fuels us, and sustains us. No diet in the world can give you that!

Chapter 2

God Can Do a New Thing in Your Fitness

"Do not remember the former things,
Nor consider the things of old. Behold, I will do a new thing,
Now it shall spring forth;
Shall you not know it? I will even make a road in the wilderness
And rivers in the desert."

Isaiah 43:18–19 NKJV

Did you know that when Moses led the Israelites out of Egypt, it took forty years to make an eleven-day trip? They circled a mountain in the wilderness for forty years.

From this example, think about how long you've been circling the mountain of trying to eat right and work out. Consider all the diets you've tried only to end up right back where you started. The Israelites were delayed their access to the Promised Land because they forgot God's promises and were obstinate and disobedient.

Some of us may not even know the promises of God. Many of us grew up unaware that we could ask Him to help us with our fitness, but God can bring us out of our wilderness and do a new thing in us. Deuteronomy 2:3 tells us: "You have circled this mountain long enough. Now turn north" (NASB).

It's important to realize that God has much more for us and that we have not arrived yet, especially if we're stuck circling a mountain of disobedience or obstinance. God wants us to know and stand on His promises. He is seeking an encounter with you. He wants you to turn to Him. In His grace, you can let go of your past attempts at getting fit, begin again, and become new in Him.

Meet Miranda

Miranda came to me because she was really struggling to get her weight down to a healthy range. She said she had tried many times to eat healthy and exercise, but she always ended up quitting, and that made her feel hopeless. Miranda had no idea that she could ask God to help her or that He cared about her desperation to get healthy. When I shared these promises with her, she said they were the life-changing help and hope she needed. They got her mindset right and gave her the strength she needed in her day-to-day life to live fit God's way.

He will never leave you or forsake you. (Deuteronomy 31:6)

God will strengthen you and uphold you. (Isaiah 41:10)

He will rescue you from every trap and protect you from deadly disease. (Psalm 91:3)

The Lord will go before you and be your rear guard. (Isaiah 52:12)

He will fight on your behalf. (Exodus 14:14)

His love will never fail you. (Isaiah 54:10)

God will give you wisdom if you ask Him. (James 1:5)

His plans are to prosper you. (Jeremiah 29:11)

God will meet all your needs according to His riches. (Philippians 4:19)

He will deliver you from all your troubles. (Psalm 34:17)

He works all things out for your good. (Romans 8:28)

He will guide and direct you. (Psalm 3:5–6)

God is your refuge and strong tower in times of trouble. (Psalm 9:9)

He will bless you and give you the crown of life. (James 1:12)

God will make you the head and not the tail. (Deuteronomy 28:13)

He will give you beauty for ashes. (Isaiah 61:3)

Grace, mercy, and peace will be with you. (2 John 1:3)

The Lord will make His face shine upon you and be gracious to you. (Numbers 6:25)

He will give you rest. (Matthew 11:28)

He has given you victory in Christ. (Romans 8:37)

In Him, you can have peace of mind and heart. (John 14:27)

You have salvation through Jesus Christ. (Romans 10:9)

He will keep His promises. (Joshua 21:45)

You have the Holy Spirit to help you. (Luke 24:49)

You have the joy of His presence. (Psalm 16:11)

You have eternal life in Him. (Romans 6:23)

With God, your sleep will be sweet. (Proverbs 3:24)

He will keep you from every disease. (Deuteronomy 7:15)

In Him, you have healing, abundant peace, and security. (Jeremiah 33:6)[1]

Friend, do you need to stand on God's promises and ask Him to do a new thing in you?

Did you know these promises are available to you? Daily, I hear from women who have no idea that God is waiting and wanting to help them. Until we confront issues that keep us from God's best, we can't experience change. Many women want to lose weight, but so often the weight they need to lose first is the weight on their hearts. The weights of rejection, the past, shame, and unforgiveness are a few examples of things that can prevent us from getting healthy. Ask God to search your heart, and let Him bring any issues to the surface. Stand on His promises, repeat them back to Him in your prayers, and let your heart be healed so He can do something new. Isaiah 55:11 says,

> "So shall My word be that goes forth from My mouth;
> It shall not return to Me void,
> But it shall accomplish what I please,
> And it shall prosper in the thing for which I sent it" (NJKV).

Here's a list of common hurts we hide in our hearts. Circle what you need to lay down in order to move forward.

- Not going to God first about my fitness and food struggles
- Guilt over gaining back all the weight I lost, and sometimes even more
- The gym memberships and workout equipment I bought and rarely used
- All the times I started a diet and quit
- Having the wrong motivation for fitness
- The foods that make me gluttonous
- Shame over the body God gave me
- Thinking that trying to be fit is hopeless
- Having unrealistic expectations
- Being lazy
- A spirit of entitlement
- Eating to numb my pain
- Holding onto weight because of past trauma
- Fear of being judged for wanting to get in great shape
- A root of bitterness, anger, or jealousy
- Believing I'm destined to be overweight or unhealthy
- Thinking it's impossible
- Body idolatry

- Making fitness an idol
- Comparing myself to others
- Thinking my value comes from how I look
- Desperately trying to lose weight to look good for an event instead of taking care of myself every day
- Not teaching my kids how to be healthy
- Keeping the clothes in my closet that I'm praying will fit me again
- The way I talk about myself so critically
- Hating the way God made my body
- Valuing my appearance more than I should
- Judging other fit women and secretly being jealous of them
- Getting sucked into overly filtered social media selfies and letting them make me feel inferior
- Thinking fitness is easier for other people and that I have it harder than they do
- The lies the enemy has made me believe about myself
- The way I've let other people make me believe I'm not good enough
- Settling for less than God's best for me
- Giving up

Now, look at the letter below and circle the things you are asking God to do in you. This is your time. Let God do a new thing in you!

Dear God,

My heart is excited and full of hope. I believe you can do a new thing in me, Lord. Please help me:

- *Believe there is victory over my fitness struggles*
- *Gain the wisdom I need over food*
- *Hit pause before I eat and invite the Holy Spirit to help me walk in self-control*

- *Rely on Your strength to work out*
- *Find motivation to take care of myself to fulfill every plan You have for my life*
- *Be brave enough to take workout classes regardless of how I look or how unfit I feel*
- *Listen to what You say about me more than anyone else*
- *See myself through Your eyes*
- *Stop falling for worldly get-fit-quick gimmicks*
- *Find confidence knowing You formed me and made me and You don't make mistakes*
- *Get free from the number on the scale, the size of my clothes, or the number of candles on my cake*
- *Know that it's not too late and I'm not too old*
- *Find peace in surrendering all of this to You daily*
- *Know I can become the woman You want me to be*

In Jesus's name, amen.

Write Yourself a "God Can Do a New Thing in Me" Letter

It's time to write a new chapter of your fitness story, but you need to cross the bridge from your old way of getting fit and feeling confident to a new way in Christ. When I was first going through a weight-loss transformation, I hit a wall of frustration. I had spent weeks eating right and working out, but the scale wasn't budging. I called a good friend and shared what I was going through. She asked me, "Have you ever written a letter to God about how hard getting fit is and asked for His help?"

> **"Blessed is she who has believed that the Lord would fulfill his promises to her!"**
> —Luke 1:45 NIV

When our call ended, I grabbed my journal, curled up on the couch, and let the words spill onto the pages along with my tears.

Prior to that rainy Saturday afternoon, I had never admitted to myself how painful and frustrating this was or how fitness had made me feel like a failure.

The words didn't lie. I didn't worry about grammar, I didn't judge myself, I just let it all out. I looked down and saw words like *hopeless, not good enough, overwhelmed,* and *frustrated.* Looking back, I know it was God's way of showing me this isn't how it's supposed to be.

We can do nothing apart from Him—so friend, hand God your pain today, take Him to the places that make you want to quit, stand on His promises, and become a new you in Him.

I challenge you to try it. Grab your journal, write your "God can do a new thing in me" letter, and watch Him work!

Fit God's Way Power-Up Plan

Power-Up Points

- God must be first in our fitness; anything we put before Him is an idol.
- Jesus is our perfect role model for living fit. Follow His ways.
- You're not alone in your fitness journey. God has left you a Helper, Counselor, and Advocate—the Holy Spirit.
- Redefine fitness God's way to put an end to the frustrating flesh project.
- Fitness is more than eating and working out: it's a battle of flesh and Spirit that worldly solutions can't answer.
- Stop circling the mountain of trying to get healthy by standing on God's promises.
- Take God to the places where you quit, the hurts that hold you back, and ask Him to do a new thing in your fitness.

Promises

"Because he loves me," says the LORD, "I will rescue him; I will protect him, for he acknowledges my name." (Psalm 91:14 NIV)

When wisdom enters your heart,
And knowledge is pleasant to your soul,
Discretion will preserve you;
Understanding will keep you,
To deliver you from the way of evil...
(Proverbs 2:10–12 NKJV)

"But when he, the Spirit of truth, comes, he will guide you into all the truth. He will not speak on his own; he will speak only what he hears, and he will tell you what is yet to come." (John 16:13 NIV)

Prayer

Dear God,
My past attempts at getting healthy have been apart from You, and they've never worked. I've struggled alone, and it has felt impossible, but what has been impossible for me is possible with You (Luke 18:27). Your Word says that "if I trust in You and acknowledge You in all my ways, You will direct my path" (Proverbs 3:5–6). Father, I'm laying down my old ways and seeking You first in my fitness (Matthew 6:33). Guide me in the Holy Spirit and give me the steps. I've gone through things that have hurt me so badly that I have felt like I can't or don't deserve to succeed, but Your Word says that "because I love You, You will rescue me" (Psalm 91:14). Father, please save me from the lies the enemy wants me to believe. Your Word says that You will do a new thing (Isaiah 43:18). Help me take each step with You, starting today, so I can be the godly woman you made me to be. In Jesus's name, amen.

HABIT 2:

Get Fit God's Way with the 7 Ws

How to Get Fit God's Way with the 7 Ws

*"Not by might, nor by power, but by my Spirit," says the
Lord of hosts.*

Zechariah 4:6 ESV

How many times have you excitedly set a fitness goal, but somehow, it
never made its way from your thoughts to your to-do list? Ninety-five
percent of the women I work with tell me they have a continuously negative
conversation going on within themselves. They share how they come to the
end of their day and have thoughts like *I know I need to spend more time
with God, I can't believe I haven't worked out this week, I need to eat
better,* and *Why can't I be consistent?* But when I ask them if they have
ever put a daily plan together, they say no!

We Can Do Nothing Apart from God

Most of us grew up learning that dieting was the only way to lose
weight, that getting fit was done apart from God, and this is why it's such
a place of struggle. The Bible tells us, "We can do nothing apart from Him."

"I am the vine, you are the branches. He who abides in Me, and
I in him, bears much fruit; for without Me you can do nothing."
(John 15:5 NKJV)

33

Ending the struggle of doing fitness in your own strength is the defining difference of Fit God's Way. Getting fit God's way means that we recognize we can do nothing apart from Him, and that because of Him, we have the gift of the Holy Spirit to help us.

Jesus promised us that because He was going to the Father, we would have the presence of the Holy Spirit. His presence is active, not passive. He isn't our silent partner; He is present and powerful, and He is producing fruit in us.

Rely on the Power of the Holy Spirit

Without God in our fitness, we're left to motivate ourselves to accomplish our goals in our own strength and for our own glory. We fuel ourselves on memes that say things like, *"Suck it up, buttercup," "Dig deeper,"* and *"The best project you'll ever work on is you."* But this type of motivation can only last for so long. When our goals are powered by self and for self, they result in inconsistency and emptiness, because God doesn't honor anything that isn't done for His glory and His purposes.

The goal of this section is to help you create a God-honoring, fit lifestyle—one that makes Him the centerpiece. It eliminates all the guesswork and gives you a solid, clear plan. This is what has been missing from your fitness. No longer will you come to the end of your day and mentally rehearse all the things you didn't do. Fit God's Way isn't just another fitness program—it will teach you to enjoy the process, grow in God, and find grace for the journey.

> **"Establish your goals with God; then He will accomplish them through you."**
> —Crystal Storms

The Apostle Paul, who wrote two-thirds of the New Testament, shares how he relied on the Holy Spirit, and we must do the same.

And my message and my preaching were very plain. Rather than using clever and persuasive speeches, I relied only on the power of the Holy Spirit. (1 Corinthians 2:4 NKJV)

Meet Marina

Marina came to me because she wanted to get serious about her health. Her doctor had warned her that she was prediabetic. Marina had tried many diets and workouts, but she had never asked God to help her. She told me she was scared.

When we went over her history together, Marina confessed that in the past, her fitness goals were just thoughts, but she never knew how to make them into a daily plan. She was confused about how to schedule workouts, eat healthy, and find the motivation. Teaching Marina the steps within this section gave her the tools she had been missing. After one month of putting them into practice, she said, "This was exactly what I needed, and I've finally found results."

Maybe today you feel like Marina, and you've never had the tools to make fitness your way of life. In this section, I'll teach you how to do that in a way that is uniquely yours. One-size-fits-all fitness plans don't work. Each of us has different goals, so we need a personalized system.

How to Make Getting Fit God's Way a Habit

To begin building the habit of getting Fit God's Way, you'll follow these steps:

1. Set F.A.I.T.H. Goals
2. Create your Fit God's Way System
3. Take the #FitGodsWay Challenge

You may be wondering why you need to set goals and create a system. The answer is, it's not enough to set a goal. We need a daily guide showing us the way to get there. Together, these create our daily system.

There are key differences between goals and systems:

F.A.I.T.H. Goals

These goals are the faith-filled, long-term healthy vision. For example, they are the pounds you want to lose, the date of the marathon on the calendar, or the mission trip you want to take. They focus on your "why" and how you're going to stay accountable.

Fit God's Way System

This system is a reverse-engineered daily action plan. It takes your big goal and breaks it into bite-sized, doable daily tasks. It clearly defines the how, when, where, and what. It helps you create small daily wins, eliminates not knowing what to do, and helps you stay the course.

Chapter 3

Set F.A.I.T.H. Goals

Then the Lord answered me and said: "Write the vision
And make it plain on tablets,
That he may run who reads it."

Habakkuk 2:2 NKJV

When I wrote *10 Steps to Your Faith Inspired Transformation, F.I.T.* in 2014, I had no idea F.A.I.T.H. Goals would transform thousands of women's lives. It was my twist on SMART Goals, which were developed in the early 1980s as a way to clarify management goals and objectives. The difference between the two is that SMART Goals don't include God, whereas F.A.I.T.H. Goals are set by seeking God first, making sure the objectives are in line with His will, and motivated by carrying out His call for your life.

> **"You are never too old to set another goal or to dream a new dream."**
> —C. S. Lewis

A sweet word of warning: whether we admit it or not, we tend to count ourselves out. We can have thoughts like *It's too late* or *I'm too old*, and these feelings produce a life that makes us feel small. Please don't do that. Remember how big our God is, and trust Him to believe again.

Proof That Writing Down Your Goals Works!

There is proof that writing down your goals helps make them a reality, and if you have an accountability partner, you double your chance of reaching them. Dr. Gail Matthews, a psychology professor at Dominican University in California, conducted a study showing that 70 percent of the participants who had written down goals and sent weekly updates to a friend either completed their objectives or were more than halfway there by the time the study ended, compared to 35 percent of those who kept their goals to themselves without writing them down.[1] Not only do I teach this and see it change women every day, I believe it and do it myself. Over the last five years, God has made these F.A.I.T.H. Goals of mine realities:

- Land a deal with a Christian publishing house and write a Bible-based book about food, fitness, and wholeness that reaches women all around the world.
- Start the *Strong. Confident. His.* podcast to reach as many women as possible for God, covering every topic necessary to help them with their food, fitness, and sense of worth.
- Create a workout for Christian women and stream it on a Christian platform.
- Build a Christian fitness ministry and host a space called F.I.T. Sisters-in-Christ for Christian women to connect, hold each other accountable, and find support.
- Write a beautiful faith and fitness devotional so women have a constant reminder of who they are in Christ.
- Be the very best wife, mother, and sister/friend I can be.
- Live Fit God's Way by practicing what I preach.

Setting goals is important to your success for these key reasons:

1. It shows you what you really want and eliminates what you don't.
2. It gets you focused and motivated.

3. It helps you achieve the plans God has for you.

Grab your journal and prayerfully seek God's heart for you in each of these areas.

Set Your F.A.I.T.H. Goals

F   Faith-Filled and Specific
A   Accountable
I   Inspiring
T   Time-Based and Measurable
H   Healthy

F. Faith-Filled and Specific

Ask God what His will is for you in your goals. It is not His will that we are unhealthy, out of shape, gluttonous, lazy, or insecure. Here are some examples of Faith-Filled and Specific goals: Read the Bible every day, lose weight, lower blood pressure, start a small faith and fitness group, work out five days a week, or eat whole, God-made foods instead of man-made, processed foods. Have a prayer meeting with God about your goal. Get excited about it and ask Him to show you His specific plan for you in this area.

A. Accountable

The best accountability you will ever have is the time you spend with God. Accountability is that daily push that gets you to your goal. Being accountable to ourselves is how we honor those self-made promises and glorify God. How will you stay accountable? Examples of accountability include: Morning prayer time with God; a trusted workout partner; an alarm that goes off on your phone when it's time to read your Bible; a food journal or app to track your daily meals, snacks, and drinks; a Christian group of women like my private Facebook Group, F.I.T. Sisters-in-Christ; signing up for an event like running or walking for a cause; or joining a challenge at your workout studio, gym, or the #FitGodsWay Challenge.

I. Inspiring

God has a plan for you, and nothing fuels your motivation to carry it out like living for Him. What dream has He given you that you've tucked away? Put pen to paper and write it down. Is it starting a new business, getting healthy to avoid diseases that run in your family, or to be a great role model for your kids? Inspiration comes from your "why." Why do you want to achieve this goal? How would your life be different if you did? What doors of opportunity would open for you? Whose lives would change if this goal were met? Collect scriptures and Christian songs to keep this motivation fresh.

T. Time-Based and Measurable

God wants us living with intention and discipline. Having a date that you're working toward helps keep you focused. Set a date of accomplishment for your goal and a method of tracking your success. If weight loss is your goal, do not use the scale as your only measure; buy a measuring tape, take pictures, or use a favorite pair of jeans that you want to fit well again. As your body remodels itself with your healthy eating and exercise, these very important changes are not always evident on the scale. An important note here is that this is a grace-based health journey, not a slave-to-numbers project, so sprinkle these measurements with grace.

> **"Set your goals high and your sights on the only One who can take you there. The hard work you do in Christ is the birthplace of your success."**
> —Kim Dolan Leto

H. Healthy

God doesn't want us living with extremes, so make sure your goal is healthy, realistic, and achievable. It's not fair of you to pressure yourself to lose thirty pounds in a month, run a marathon after a week of training, or know how to cook all your food in a healthy way after a week or two. Remember, this is a process, and the joy is found in the journey.

All too often, our goals never become more than a thought, a wish written on a page of our journals or a sticky note on our desk. But F.A.I.T.H Goals make God the centerpiece of our fitness; they help us envision who He made us to be and put the date on the calendar. The Fit God's Way System is how we take our F.A.I.T.H. Goals and break them into the daily steps we must take to achieve them.

SET YOUR F.A.I.T.H. GOALS WORKSHEET

F - Faith-Filled and Specific

_____

_____

_____

A - Accountable

_____

_____

_____

I - Inspiring

_____

_____

_____

T - Time-Based and Measurable

_____

_____

_____

H - Healthy

_____

_____

_____

Chapter 4

The 7 Ws: Your Fit God's Way System

Unless the Lord builds the house,
They labor in vain who build it.

Psalm 127:1 NKJV

In the beginning of this book, I invited you to take the #FitGodsWay Challenge. This challenge is based on the 7 Ws, which are explained here in depth. This section will help you go deeper, teach you how to create your personal system of success for your goals, and make Fit God's Way a lifestyle for you.

Your Fit God's Way System is the daily working application of the 7 Habits you will learn. They take the guesswork out of how to reach your F.A.I.T.H. Goals by putting a daily system together. This system answers the *what, when, where,* and *how* of achieving your goals.

The Fit God's Way Daily System: The 7 Ws
(Print weekly template at www.fitgodsway.com)
Word: Read your Bible and pray.
Worth: Practice placing your worth in Christ to find confidence, strength, and grace.
Whole, God-Made Food: Choose whole, God-made food over

man-made, processed foods. Focus on quality ingredients versus obsessing over quantities. Pray before meals.

Water: Divide your weight in half and drink a minimum of that many ounces per day. Add seven to ten ounces of fluid every ten to twenty minutes during exercise.

Work Out: Move and strengthen your body five to six days a week. Increase your non-exercise activity calorie burn by taking walks outdoors to spend time in God's creation and mini-movement breaks throughout the day.

Worship: Listen to Christian music, sing, dance, and praise God.

Wake/Sleep: Establish a wake/sleep cycle and a morning/evening routine to put yourself to bed in the peace of God and wake up in His power.

The 7 Ws Explained

Here is a breakdown of each of the Ws and tips to help you start building your Fit God's Way System.

Word

Habit One teaches the importance of getting into the Word daily.

> "This Book of the Law shall not depart from your mouth, but you shall meditate in it day and night, that you may observe to do according to all that is written in it. For then you will make your way prosperous, and then you will have good success." (Joshua 1:9 NKJV)

Spending time with God is the most important part of your day. Jesus got up early and spent time with His Father, and we should do the same. Instead of starting your diet over every Monday, have a morning meeting with God instead. Get up and talk to Him, surrender your goals to Him, and ask Him to help you honor Him in your body. Doing this every day is the best way to stay connected to Him, and it helps you rededicate your goals to make fitness a Spirit-led lifestyle—not just another fleeting attempt at getting healthy.

From Him, to Him, and *through Him,* you will be able to do the things you think you cannot do. When we allow days without time in the Word to slip by, they often turn into weeks and even months. Our time with Him is our truest strength training and our first priority. If you can only get one W in all day, this is the one you don't want to miss!

There is a beautiful hymn called "Give Me Jesus" which says, "In the morning, when I rise, give me Jesus." This is the way to start every day! Make your time in the Word a daily habit, and you will see God work all things for your good. With that in mind, fill out the following:

When will you read your Bible and pray?

Where will you read your Bible?

Will you follow a Bible plan for reading? If so, which one?

How will you remind yourself to pray before meals,

workouts, sleep, and throughout the day?

Tips

- If you're just starting out and don't know where to start reading the Bible, there are many reading plans available. Do an internet search for "Bible reading plans," select one to follow, and keep it in your Bible.
- Get a Bible app on your phone.
- Subscribe to a verse-of-the-day app.
- It's best to set a time every day to read your Bible and stick to it. Getting alone in the morning is a great time to read the Word before you get busy. Another great time is at night right before bed. If you're a busy working mom and neither of these times work, get the Bible on audiobook and listen while you

drive to work, run errands, and wait for your kids in the pickup line at school.

- Remember, God wants a relationship with you, so this isn't a to-do list where you just check off "time with God." I believe God would rather you read one verse, spend time meditating on it, and seek His heart for you than speed-read a full chapter to get your check mark for the day.
- Prayer is powerful, so find times throughout the day to pray. Here are some examples: before you get out of bed, before meals, before and after your workout, while you're on a walk, before bed, and with your family.

Worth

Habit Two covers worthiness in depth.

> You know how we exhorted and comforted...every one of you...that you would walk worthy of God who calls you into His own kingdom and glory. (1 Thessalonians 2:11–12 NKJV)

The mindset you have about your worth is determining the course of your life. This mindset either says *I'm worthy to reach my goals* or *I'm unworthy*. It's important to take hold of the gift that God has given you. Christ died for you. He took every sin you've ever committed or will commit in the future, and He paid for it. Walk in that freedom. He chose you. He set you apart. He has a perfect plan for you, so throughout your day, speak His truth over yourself and your fitness. Practice spotting the things that rob you of your confidence, your peace, or your passion, and remember that you are worthy because He is worthy.

When do you need to practice telling yourself, "I'm worthy, I'm good enough, because He is more than enough"?

Where are the places or situations in your life that you need to remind yourself that you are worthy?

What is standing between you and your worthiness?

How will you remind yourself throughout the day to practice worthiness in Christ?

Tips

- If you struggle with body image, practice looking in the mirror and inhaling as you say, "I'm enough." As you exhale say, "Because He is enough."
- If you struggle with past sin, write down the word *tetelestai*, and then write it across your heart. "*Tetelestai*" was the last thing Jesus said on the cross. It means "it is finished." It was written on documents in New Testament times to say "paid in full." Our sins have been paid in full. There is nothing we can do to earn it—it is a free gift. "If we confess our sins, He is faithful and just to forgive us our sins and to cleanse us from all unrighteousness" (1 John 1:9 NKJV). Guilt is our way of trying to pay for what God has already done. Lay it at His feet, and let Him lift you up.
- If you feel like you're not good enough because of what someone else has done to you or said about you, take your power back by extending to them the same forgiveness that God has given you.
- Put an alert on your phone with a scripture to remind yourself of your worth in Christ.
- Think of the common situations that make you question your worth. Learn a go-to Bible verse you can speak over these times and pray back to God.

Whole, God-Made Foods

Habit Three comprehensively teaches about whole, God-made foods.

"Every moving thing that lives shall be food for you. I have given you all things, even as the green herbs." (Genesis 9:3 NKJV)

Fit God's Way is not a diet, it is a Spirit-led lifestyle that teaches intentional eating; forming a healthy relationship with food; and choosing God-made, whole foods over man-made, processed foods. Habit Three is dedicated to equipping you with everything you need to know—but for now, begin to pray about these questions and choose whole, God-made foods over man-made, processed foods.

When will you plan your meals, shop for groceries, do your meal prep, and cook?

Where can you eat out? Which restaurants serve whole, God-made foods?

What man-made, processed foods can you replace with healthy, God-made foods?

What will you do if you overindulge? (Hint: skip the guilt, and get back on track in grace.)

Who will benefit from your healthier cooking?

How will you handle cravings, emotions, parties, and weekends?

Tips

- If eating God-made food is new to you, don't get overwhelmed. Take one step at a time. For example: replace your sodas with iced tea or sparkling mineral water, trade your burger and fries for a grilled chicken sandwich on whole-grain bread, or exchange your mid-afternoon sugary snack with half of an apple and a tablespoon of nut butter.
- Try one thing at a time. Start with your drinks, then move on to healthier side dishes, then healthier main dishes, and then try prep cooking a meal or two in advance.

- Get familiar with labels. If you can't pronounce it, and it sounds more like chemicals than food, you probably shouldn't eat it.
- Start to look for ways to replace the man-made foods you eat with healthier, God-made choices.
- Begin to collect recipes of your favorite foods with whole, God-made ingredients.

Water

The Spirit and the bride say, "Come!" And let the one who hears say, "Come!" Let the one who is thirsty come; and let the one who wishes take the free gift of the water of life. (Revelation 22:17 NIV)

Isn't it something that the Bible mentions water 722 times? Jesus is our spiritual water. He is referred to as our living water. We need Him for our spiritual health, and we need water for our physical and mental health. Water is a gift, and our bodies need it to function. Did you know that your body is 60 percent water?

Here are some signs of not getting enough water: fatigue, digestive issues, and headaches.

God gave us the gift of water. To help you drink more of it, prayerfully reframe water as a gift from Him and a necessity for your body's health.

When will you drink water?

Where will you keep your water? For example, a sports bottle or glass jar?

What drinks need to be replaced with water?

How will you keep track of how much water you drink each day?

Tips

If you currently don't drink as much water as you should, here is a guideline to help: Drink it when you wake up; before, during, and after workouts; and before you eat, while you eat, and after you eat. Keep a BPA-free bottle with you for drinking throughout the day. BPA stands for bisphenol A, an industrial chemical that has been used to make certain plastics and resins since the 1950s, which is linked to several health concerns.[1]

If you are looking for healthy ways to flavor your water:

- Add fruit slices, particularly lemon, lime, or orange.
- Infuse water with berries.
- Try cucumber slices with basil or mint.
- Love your bubbles? Try sparkling water.

If you don't know how much water to drink, start by taking your weight and dividing it in half to determine the number of ounces you should be drinking.

Work Out

Habit Five teaches you how to do fitness through faith.

> Or do you not know that your body is the temple of the Holy Spirit who is in you, whom you have from God, and you are not your own? For you were bought at a price; therefore glorify God in your body and in your spirit, which are God's. (1 Corinthians 6:19–20 NKJV)

God calls us to take care of our bodies. Treat workouts like appointments, and mark off the time for them in your day. Moving and strengthening your body gives you the energy and ability to carry out His plans for you. Begin to consider the internal health benefits of your workouts versus focusing on aesthetics. The external results will come with time and consistency, so be patient; fitness is an inside-out process. Stewarding our bodies in a manner that honors God is our goal.

What days and times will you work out?

Which workout will you do? Which scriptures will you take with you?
What will you do if you get bored?
What workouts can you do at home in case your kids get sick,
the class gets canceled, etc.?
Where will you work out?
How long will you work out?

Tips

- Begin to see fitness as a way of honoring God with your body.
- Notice the benefits of working out apart from what you look like, such as less stress, better sleep, improved mood, or more confidence. Let those things fuel your motivation.
- Invite a friend to work out with you. This will help you stay accountable.
- Know that you don't have to choose a one-size-fits all workout program. You can take a group fitness class, sign up for a walkathon, take up cycling, etc.
- If you'd like a faith-based workout you can do at home, try my *Faith-Inspired Transformation Workout* on Pure Flix.
- Listen to a Christian playlist while you work out. (Try mine for free on Spotify.)
- Listen to the Bible and Christian podcasts while you work out. My podcast *Strong. Confident. His.* will motivate and inspire you with faith-filled tips and prayer for your fitness journey.
- Share your workouts on social media to inspire others.
- Challenge yourself by taking the #FitGod'sWay Challenge to jumpstart your new Spirit-led fit lifestyle.

Worship

Habits One and Six teach about dedicating our fitness to God.

And so, dear brothers and sisters, I plead with you to give your bodies to God because of all he has done for you. Let them be a living and holy sacrifice—the kind he will find acceptable. This is truly the way to worship him. (Romans 12:1 NLT)

Did you know the Bible mentions worship 8,629 times? Believers are called to worship. Worshipping God is a powerful part of the Christian life. Worship is showing God you love Him with all of your heart, mind, soul, and strength, and living a life of obedience to His commandments.

When we worship God, we come into His presence, and we give Him honor and praise. The Bible shares many examples of what happens when His followers worship Him. Drawing closer to Him strengthens our faith and enables us to live from a place of peace and victory. Studies have also shown that it lowers stress, reduces physical pain, and increases joy and love for others. Worship is at the beginning of most church services, so make time to participate in it.

When will you worship God?

Where will you worship God?

What music and/or activity helps you worship?

How will you worship God more throughout your day?

Tips

- Don't overthink it. Worshipping God is as easy as putting on your favorite worship playlist as you drive. Create a worship playlist to make this a regular part of your day.
- To worship God is to serve Him, so look for opportunities to serve, volunteer, and donate.
- Worship God by praying His Word back to Him.
- From home: sing, raise your hands, or get down on your knees and praise Him.

Wake/Sleep

"Come to me, all you who are weary and burdened, and I will give you rest. Take my yoke upon you and learn from me, for I am gentle and humble in heart, and you will find rest for your souls. For my yoke is easy and my burden is light." (Mark 11:28–30 NIV)

Our culture doesn't place a lot of value on resting, but the Bible sure does. Many of us are tired and stressed from not getting enough sleep. One of the best things you can do to reach your fitness goals is to rest. Inadequate sleep causes the stress hormone cortisol to rise, which can lead to increased body fat in our midsections. Poor sleep contributes to heart disease, diabetes, and mood disorders. The body needs seven to nine hours of sleep. Did you know muscles do all their repairing in rest? And the more muscle we carry, the more calories we burn throughout the day—even while sleeping—and that leads to greater overall fat loss and better health. So establishing a consistent sleep schedule and wake/sleep routine is one of the best ways to take care of yourself.

When will you wake up and go to sleep? Create consistent sleep and wake times.

Where do you need to discipline yourself to make sleep a priority? For example, what time will you turn off your phone, TV, or laptop?

Which Scriptures can you pray back to God to help you sleep well?

How will you wind down? Get up? Create nightly routines and morning routines.

Tips

- Turn off your phone and eliminate blue light for two to three hours before bed; it hinders the sleep hormone melatonin from functioning, causing poor sleep.

- Before sleep, prepare for the next day by doing a brain dump. This will help you avoid lying in bed and ruminating over your to-do list.
- Pray right before sleep and right when you wake up.
- Morning routines set the tone of the day—so instead of turning on the TV or your phone, open your Bible, enjoy your coffee or tea, and go over your plan for the day.

How to Get Started with Your 7 Ws

There are many ways to start adding the 7 Ws into your life. Look at these guidelines so you won't feel overwhelmed, pressured to be perfect, or think you can't do it—because in Him, you can!

Pray over the 7 Ws and fill out the template in the appendix. Ask God to guide you.

Start small. If the 7 Ws feel overwhelming, choose one W to focus on for a week, and then build on it by adding another W the next week. Slow and steady always wins the race.

Go all in. If fitness is already a part of your life and you want to do it God's way, aim to get in all of the 7 Ws.

Invest in your health and wholeness fearlessly. This may be new to you, so don't worry, feel intimidated, or be insecure. If you don't know how to do a W, this book will teach you; but if you still need more help, you'll find it at www.fitgodsway.com.

Acknowledge small wins. Celebrate the Ws you get in by thanking God, sharing with a friend, or posting about them on social media.

Choose grace over perfection. This is not a worldly perfection project. If you miss a day, or you just want to do three of the 7 Ws, congratulations! You are building a foundation of fitness through faith. Do the best you can, and God will bless your efforts.

Remember you have an enemy. The devil doesn't want you focused on honoring God in your body, getting healthier, or feeling whole. He will try to derail you with doubt, negativity, and comparison. Learn to spot the things that discourage you, and don't take the bait!

Create built-in accountability. Don't go this alone. Invite a friend, start a small group, or have your family do it with you.

Rest! A complete day of rest is biblical and vital to avoiding burnout.

Take the social media #FitGodsWay Challenge to stir yourself up and share the difference God is making in your fitness. Tell the world you are getting Fit God's Way.

Here's how: Post a picture of yourself doing one or all of the 7 Ws with "#FitGodsWay" on social media. If you're wondering how to get started, here are some simple ideas:

- Take a picture of yourself praying or reading your Bible.
- Share how you find worth in Christ through favorite Scriptures, quotes, and even grace when you miss it.
- Share images of yourself eating God-made food and drinking water out of your go-to container.
- Snap a photo of yourself working out and listening to your favorite worship song, and share how you do your morning and evening routine.

Real-Life, Easy Examples of How to Get in Your 7 Ws

- Go for a walk and listen to the Word. Tune in to either the Bible, a church message, or a podcast. Worship God while you listen by thanking Him for all He's done and the beauty of nature around you. And don't forget to drink your water.
- While you prep and cook whole, God-made foods, enjoy some good

"You'll never change your life until you change something you do daily. The secret of your success is found in your daily routine."

—John C. Maxwell

praise and worship music, and enjoy some water with cucumber or lemon slices.

- Bring the Word and your water to your workout. Practice worthiness by putting scriptures on your phone or on note cards, and pray them over any insecurities you may be feeling in the moment.
- Create a wake/sleep routine of prayer and time in the Word. Give God your worries and anxieties, avoid distractions, and focus fully on Him. Worship in the last moments before you fall sleep to relax your mind and heart.
- Worship God while you work out with a Christian playlist. When you're done, enjoy some water and say a prayer before you eat a whole, God-made snack.
- Practice worthiness with your children. Teach them to see themselves through God's eyes, and pray the Word over them before you drop them off at school.
- Break up your day by getting outside and going for a walk while you listen to your favorite Christian worship music.
- Practice worthiness by writing the Word out on sticky notes and putting them on your mirror.
- Wake up, get in the Word, and enjoy a whole, God-made breakfast before you work out.
- Please share how you're getting in your 7 Ws with the #FitGodsWay on social media.

Chapter 5

Accountability, Support, and Community

*Therefore encourage one another and build one another up,
just as you are doing.*

1 Thessalonians 5:11 ESV

Accountability is an important part of the Christian life—including our health and wholeness. We're accountable to God, to others, and to ourselves for our choices and actions. Our lives are designed by the actions we decide to take or not take. Accountability is like having an insurance policy. It's that trusted Christian friend who calls you to say, "Meet me at the gym tomorrow morning early so we can pray before we work out," or even being the friend someone can call to encourage them to keep going when they want to quit.

"As iron sharpens iron, so one person sharpens another."
—Proverbs 27:17 NIV

Accountability will help you reach your goals. Without it, it's not impossible to reach them, but it will be harder. I recently had an opportunity to see how valuable accountability is. A good friend reached out to me and asked where she could find support from Christian women on her fitness journey. As we spoke, I felt a stirring within me to start a small group.

Later that week, I reached out to a few women and asked them if they'd like to be a part of a small Fit God's Way group. The goal would be to meet weekly, stay accountable throughout the week, and pray for each other daily. The response was overwhelming. The first night, I began the discussion with this question, "What has been missing from your fitness journey?"

As hands went up, I heard the following:

- I don't feel like I have any support.
- I feel really awkward going to work out alone.
- I don't have anyone to talk to about my body-image struggle.
- My hormones! Is there any help for me? Does anyone else feel like it's impossible to lose weight?
- I don't feel like anyone understands how hard it is for me to put on workout clothes when I look the way I do. I'm embarrassed about how I've let myself go.
- I'm busy taking care of everyone else. I've stopped taking care of myself.
- I don't know what to do, and I'm so confused by all the different information.
- I wish I had a friend to work out with and pray with afterward.
- I wish I had women around me who encouraged me to keep going when I want to quit.
- I don't even know where to start.
- I think I'd work out more if I had a friend to go with me.
- I want someone I can call and share my workout and recipes with so we can celebrate this lifestyle together.
- It would be so nice to have friends over and cook healthy food together.

Support, accountability, and fellowship were the topics that came up over and over again, sometimes through tears. What became obvious is that fitness and body image are deep places of struggle and pain for women, and we cannot do this alone. We need each other. So as you begin your Fit God's Way journey, don't go it alone—invite a friend or friends, start a small group, and join my private Facebook group, F.I.T. Sisters-in-Christ.

Create Accountability to Ensure Your Fit God's Way Success

- Take the #FitGodsWay Challenge, and invite a friend or friends to do it with you.
- Announce your goals on social media, share your journey, and encourage others.
- Keep your F.A.I.T.H. goals in view. Make them your phone lock screen, your screen saver, or print them out and put them on your refrigerator.
- Print out your Fit God's Way System, fill it out completely, and commit to it.
- Keep your workouts like you would doctor's appointments.
- Meet with a friend weekly to take measurements and weigh in, send each other your food and workout journals, or share each other's profiles on fitness apps.
- Don't follow the advice of anyone who isn't following Jesus. Diet pills, quick fixes, and body-part photos are not the roads to a better you. Keep your eyes on God, and become His best version of you!
- Create your own small group to encourage others and enjoy built-in accountability. Becoming a mentor, small group leader, or coach will not only help others, but will help you reach your goals.
- "Two are better than one, because they have a good reward for their toil. For if they fall, one will lift up his fellow. But

woe to him who is alone when he falls and has not another to lift him up!" (Ecclesiastes 4:9–10 ESV)

Fit God's Way Power-Up Plan

Power-Up Points

- We can do nothing apart from God, including fitness. Most of us grew up believing that dieting was the only way to lose weight and getting fit was done apart from God, and this is why it's such a place of struggle.
- We make getting fit God's way a habit by relying on the power of the Holy Spirit.
- We set F.A.I.T.H. Goals to make God the centerpiece of our fitness; they help us envision who He made us to be and put the date on the calendar. The Fit God's Way System is how we break our F.A.I.T.H. Goals into the daily steps necessary to achieve them.
- We stay accountable because accountability is vital to our success. It's like having an insurance policy. It's that trusted Christian friend who calls you to say, "Meet me at the gym tomorrow early so we can pray before we work out," or even being the friend someone can call to encourage them to keep going when they want to quit.

Promises

Make me to know your ways, O Lord;
teach me your paths.
Lead me in your truth and teach me,

for you are the God of my salvation;
for you I wait all the day long. (Psalm 25:4–6 ESV)

This is the day the Lord has made; We will rejoice and be glad in it. (Psalm 188:24 NKJV)

I can do all things through Christ who gives me strength. (Philippians 4:13 BSB)

Prayer

Dear God,

Guide me as I set goals and create a system for my fitness with You at the center of it all. My time with You is the rock on which I will build my new habits, and it will give me the strength training I need for each day. I know I can do nothing apart from You (John 15:5), but I can do all things in Your strength (Philippians 4:13). You know the goals of my heart, but the daily details are a challenge to accomplish. Let Your Spirit within me be louder than my excuses, and show me the importance of faithfulness over every small choice throughout my day. Your Word says that "the faithful over the little rule over much" (Matthew 25:23). Help me know how to "apply my heart to your instruction, and my ears to hear your words of knowledge" (Proverbs 23:12) and take action. Please bring the right strong Christian woman into my life to support me on this journey. In Jesus's name, amen.

Power-Up Challenge

Get Fit God's Way with the Daily 7 Ws

(Print weekly template at www.fitgodsway.com)

Word: Read your Bible and pray.

Worth: Practice placing your worth in Christ to find confidence, strength, and grace.

Whole, God-Made Food: Choose whole, God-made food over man-made, processed foods. Focus on quality ingredients versus obsessing over quantities. Pray before meals.

Water: Divide your weight in half and drink a minimum of that many ounces per day. Add seven to ten ounces of fluid every ten to twenty minutes during exercise.

Work Out: Move and strengthen your body five to six days a week. In addition, take walks outdoors to spend time in God's creation and mini-movement breaks throughout the day to increase your non-exercise activity calorie burn.

Worship: Listen to Christian music, sing, dance, and praise God.

Wake/Sleep: Establish a wake/sleep cycle and a morning/evening routine to put yourself to bed in the peace of God and wake up in His power.

HABIT 3:
Activate Your Faith

How to Activate Your Faith

*And hope does not put us to shame, because God's love has been poured
into our hearts through the Holy Spirit who has been given to us.*

Romans 5:5 NKJV

The power we need to accomplish our Fit God's Way 7 Ws is found in
the habit of activating our faith.

There's a scene in *The Chosen* where Simon (Peter) lets the nets down
again after a long night of fishing; in doing this, he is showing active faith.
He is tired, weary, and hopeless, but Jesus tells him to let his nets down
again, and this time they come up overflowing.

This beautiful story of active faith sets the stage for our own.

When it comes to your eating, your workouts, or dealing with the issues
that hold you back in life, do you need to let down your net again? Do you
need to believe one more time? Do you need to act in faith, without
doubting, even when reality says the possibility of a full net is just a long,
exhausting night away?

Let me rephrase this in fitness terms:

- Do you need to believe when you make healthy food choices
  that you're creating the results you want?

- Do you need to believe your workouts are working?
- Do you need to act in faith without doubting, even when nothing in reality says the possibility of your goals are just around the corner?

All too often we are unmotivated and hopeless, and this begs the question: How do we get into action? How do we pull ourselves up and out of the pits of our lives—the couch that calls our name, the workouts we wish we'd done, the healthy meals we promise to learn to cook? I hope you don't miss the connection that letting down our nets means we believe God even when we aren't seeing results. We act again to bring the results!

"Master, we've toiled all night and caught nothing; nevertheless at Your word I will let down the net." (Luke 5:5 NKJV)

"Nevertheless, at Your word I will let down the net." Luke shows us how acts of faith are rewarded. Luke 5:6–7 goes on to say, "And when they had done this, they caught a great number of fish, and their net was breaking. So they signaled to their partners in the other boat to come and help them. And they came and filled both the boats, so that they began to sink."

When the Lord is in it, there is no limit. Peter and the other disciples were astonished, and their expectations were exceeded. Jesus knew what Peter needed, and He knows exactly what we need to let down our nets again.

Activating our faith requires believing in what we do not see.

Now faith is being sure of what we hope for and certain of what we do not see.... And without faith it is impossible to please God, because anyone who comes to him must believe that he exists and that he rewards those who earnestly seek him. (Hebrews 11:1, 6 NIV)

Activate your faith with these inspiring quotes:

"You don't have to see the whole staircase, just take the first step."
—Martin Luther King Jr.

"Don't dig up in doubt what you planted in faith."
—Elisabeth Elliot

"When you can see the invisible, you can do the impossible."
—Oral Roberts

Chapter 6

The Activate-Your-Faith Success Equation

The Apostle Paul wrote that faith without works is dead (James 2:20). It's not enough to believe and pray then do nothing; we must follow up by taking actions.

> But be doers of the Word, and not hearers only, deceiving yourselves. (James 1:22 NKJV)

Some tough love here: are your actions taking you to your goals?

Meet Carissa

My client, Carissa, was a follow-through type of girl. She always did what she said she was going to do—except when it came to fitness. She worked hard, she loved her family, and she did all she could for them. Carissa had a beautiful gift for hospitality. So why was she so successful in all of these areas but not fitness?

Over coffee, she confessed to me that she felt extreme disappointment in herself from failing at her fitness goals. As the tears streamed down her face, I asked her how she was able to entertain with such ease, lovingly serve her family, and excel at work. After a long pause, she looked up and said, "Because I know I can't do it, but I know God can...I rely on Him, and He helps me do what I know I cannot do."

I said, "Aha!" We smiled at each other as she realized she needed to do the same thing with her fitness. We laughed, but it was a life-changing moment for her.

Maybe like Carissa, you find yourself very disciplined and successful in some areas of your life, but it's been a struggle to apply your strengths to your fitness goals.

The Activate-Your-Faith Success Equation: The 3 Ss

On your fitness journey, you will encounter places of struggle. Whether it's with your eating, working out, or motivation, in these difficult situations, you will need to Activate Your Faith to beat it. Here is a very helpful tool that I created from a lot of prayer.

The Activate-Your-Faith Success Equation = Seek God + Surrender it daily to God + Show up in the Spirit

Overcome your place of struggle by:

- Seeking God's wisdom for you in this area
- Surrendering it daily to God and relying on His guidance, timing, and strength
- Showing up daily in the power of Holy Spirit and owning your part

Let's break this apart and look at each one of the three Ss: Seek, Surrender, and Show Up.

Seek

We activate our faith when we seek God first. So if you're trying to find the right weight-loss program, the right workout, or the secret to confidence, make sure you're not seeking answers apart from God.

Take your battle to Him and begin to seek Him in prayer about everything, including what He made your body to eat and which foods it thrives on. In the midst of your emotions and excuses, seek God, that He might steady you; heal your pain from past fitness failures; and calm your confusion, fears, and anxieties. As we learn to seek Him for our fitness goals, He will show us the "how-to" and give us the "want-to."

Seek Scriptures

- "But seek first the kingdom of God and His righteousness, and all these things shall be added to you." (Matthew 6:33 NKJV)
- "I love those who love me. And those who seek me diligently will find me." (Proverbs 8:17 NKJV)
- "You will seek me and find me, when you seek me with all your heart." (Jeremiah 29:13 NKJV)
- Seek the Lord and His strength; seek His presence continually. (1 Chronicles 16:11 ESV)
- But if from there you seek the Lord your God, you will find him if you seek him with all your heart and with all your soul. (Deuteronomy 4:29 NIV)

Surrender

Surrendering our goals to God means we acknowledge that He is ultimately in control of everything, including our fitness goals, food struggles, and body-image issues. Daily surrender helps us let go of our expectations and whatever has been holding us back from God's best for our lives.

Surrender Scriptures

- "Be still, and know that I am God . . ." (Psalm 46:10 NKJV)
- A man's heart plans his way, but the LORD directs his steps. (Proverbs 16:9 NKJV)
- The steps of a good man are ordered by the LORD, and He delights in his way. (Psalm 37:23 NKJV)
- Therefore submit to God. Resist the devil and he will flee from you. (James 4:7 NKJV)
- Humble yourselves in the sight of the Lord, and He will lift you up. (James 4:10 NKJV)

Show Up

Showing up means we own our part by getting in our Fit God's Way 7 Ws. We take action and authority to overcome excuses and laziness. We rely on the power of the Holy Spirit working in us rather than our own weak willpower.

Show-Up Scriptures

- I can do all things through Christ who strengthens me. (Philippians 4:13 NKJV)
- Do you not know that those who run in a race all run, but one receives the prize? Run in such a way that you may obtain it. (1 Corinthians 9:24 NKJV)
- Commit your work to the Lord, and your plans will be established. (Proverbs 16:3 ESV)
- Whatever you do, work heartily, as for the Lord and not for men. (Colossians 3:23 ESV)
- Delight yourself in the LORD, and he will give you the desires of your heart. (Psalm 37:4 ESV)

- [Y]ou have put off the old self with its practices and have put on the new self, which is being renewed in knowledge after the image of its creator. (Colossians 3:9–10 ESV)

Where do you need to Seek God, Surrender to Him, and Show Up in the Holy Spirit to activate your faith?

- Is it making healthy meals or eating smaller portions?
- Is it making movement and workouts a habit?
- Is it making fitness more about taking care of your body than obsessing over trying to make it look a certain way?

Activating our faith leads us to success, which is satisfying, deep, and liberating. Consider writing down what being successful at fitness would look like for you without worldly ideals. For example, a Godly definition of fitness success might be: Because of God's love for me, I'm worth the best care I can give myself. Regardless of how I look, I choose to nourish and exercise my body toward godliness. I want to be fit in my mind, body, and soul to accomplish every good thing God planned for me long ago.

"When I stand before God at the end of my life, I would hope that I would not have a single bit of talent left but could say I've used everything you gave me."
—Erma Bombeck

Chapter 7

Tools to Help You
Take Action

I once heard someone jokingly say, "You have to put your toe in the Red Sea for God to part the waters." As I studied Exodus in the Old Testament, I learned that God actually told Moses, "Why are you crying out to me? Tell the people to get moving!" (Exodus 14:15 NLT)

It gave me a completely new perspective on how God is waiting on us to act. For a moment, picture God saying to you, "Why are you crying to Me? Get moving!" Because this is exactly what we must do. It's in our doing that He can help us.

You know what this whole book comes down to? Acting in faith. Active faith isn't just believing—it's moving, it's doing, it's pushing yourself, and it's knowing if you do your part, God is doing His!

It doesn't matter how long you've been where you are or how impossible your goals seem: God wants you to get up and live for Him!

Think of the paralytic man in John 5:6–9 who sat next to the healing pool in Bethesda for thirty-eight years.

When Jesus saw him lying there and learned that he had been in this condition for a long time, he asked him, "Do you want to get well?"

"Sir," the invalid replied, "I have no one to help me into the pool when the water is stirred. While I am trying to get in, someone else goes down ahead of me." Then Jesus said to him, "Get up! Pick up your mat and walk." At once the man was cured; he picked up his mat and walked. (NIV)

Picture Jesus asking you, "Do you want to get well?" What would you say? What are you doing about it? Surely this man could've gotten in the water at some point, but he didn't. What held him back? What's holding you back?

Jesus is telling us through this story, "Get up! Pick up your beds and walk."

When I think of the bed this man laid on all those years, I can't help but think about the comfortable beds of excuses, laziness, or fear we make for ourselves. But God is saying, "Get up!" When the man got up, he was healed. Can you imagine the joy he felt? The freedom to be able to walk? If we get up in Christ, we can pull ourselves up and out of the issues that paralyze us and live with joy, too!

Getting into action means we override our feelings with God's greater purpose. This is not easy stuff when we live in a world where you can have DoorDash bring donuts to your house.

Three Tools to Help You Take Action

The Five-Second Rule

One morning, my husband and I were eating breakfast when he started telling me about a tool he was using to help him get up from his desk and go work out: The Five-Second Rule, developed by author and speaker Mel Robbins.

Robbins explains, "If you have an instinct to act on a goal, you must physically move within five seconds, or your brain will kill it."

The moment you feel an instinct or a desire to act on a goal or a commitment, use this rule. When you feel yourself hesitate before doing something you know you should do, count 5, 4, 3, 2, 1, GO, and move toward the action.[1]

One of the biggest battles faced by the women who ask me for help is getting into action. I decided to try the five-second rule for myself, and I have to admit, there's something to it.

You know those cold mornings when the last thing in the world you want to do is pry yourself from the warmth and comfort of your bed to get up early to read your Bible, make a healthy breakfast, or go work out? I've put this five-second rule and a scripture into my morning routine, and now it gets me on my feet. As I open my eyes, I say, "This is the day the Lord has made. I will rejoice and be glad in it, 5, 4, 3, 2, 1, get up!"

I know it sounds very simple, but if there's a point in your day when you start to talk yourself out of doing any of the 7 Ws, try it. Rather than beginning a conversation with yourself that ultimately talks you out of what you really want to do, try 5, 4, 3, 2, 1, GO, and see if it helps you, too.

Win the Moment in Front of You

Do your fitness goals feel so impossible and far away that the feeling of defeat overrides wanting to do your best today?

Think about it. What fitness goal are you going after? Does it feel like losing twenty pounds in three months will just take too long? Winning the moment in front of you is how you can reframe it from something that feels impossible to a bite-sized step you can take now! The idea of creating small wins to win the day is powerful, because it takes the focus from how big and overwhelming your goal can feel to a clear winning step you can take today.

Mark Batterson is one of my favorite authors. In his book *Win the Day*, he writes:

What impossible problem are you trying to solve, what unbreakable habit are you trying to change, what God-sized goal are you going after? While the win may be defined differently for each of us the secret to success remains the same, it all starts with this one simple question: Can you do it for a day?[2]

Which begs the questions:

- Can you read your Bible for a day?
- Can you work out for a day?
- Can you choose God-made foods for a day?
- Can you see yourself as fearfully and wonderfully made for a day?
- Can you press on and not quit for a day?

Fitness is filled with ups and downs, so we need to continually direct our attention back to God. He wants us to live fully present with Him in each moment—not in the past or in the future, but in the nowness of life! Winning the moment in front of us is how we keep our focus and reach big goals—one small win at a time.

I think we forget to celebrate the impossible things that God is doing in the now. When we look back, we see all He's brought us through. We long for miracles in the future, but He's watching our faithfulness in the now, and it is determining our course.

> Jesus replied, "What is impossible with man is possible with God." (Luke 18:27 NIV)

We set our goals with excitement, but over time, our motivation can fade and make us want to quit. Take a moment to think about an impossible circumstance God brought you through. Let it serve as a reminder that He can do the impossible in you. In the in-between places, God wants us to be faithful and praise Him like it's already done. In our moments of frustration, impatience, and complaining, let's begin to choose to win the moment in front of us! I love the saying, "Until God answers the door, praise Him in the hallway." Let's reframe it for our fitness goals: "Until God helps me reach my goal, I'll praise Him with this small win!"

Habit Stacking

Did you know your whole day is a series of habits, and your life is a product of those habits? Think about it: do you tell yourself to brush your teeth, make coffee, or drive to work? We do so much on autopilot. And this gives us unbelievable hope, because we can train ourselves to create the habits we really want. Building on the habits we already have is called habit stacking, a concept I learned from author James Clear's book *Atomic Habits*, where he explains, "The habit stacking formula is: After [Current Habit], I will [New Habit]."[3]

Consider the 7 Ws and the habits you're trying to build into your life as you read this quote he is famous for: "You do not rise to the level of your goals. You fall to the level of your systems. Decide the type of person you want to be. Prove it to yourself with small wins." When we develop the seven habits of putting God first in our fitness, applying the Fit God's Way 7 Ws, activating our faith, choosing fit thoughts, eating to fuel our temples, working out God's way, and pressing on, we can live in victory over our fitness!

I've taught habit stacking to many women, and I've learned that we are multitaskers who also follow our own version of habit stacking. For us, it's more like "While I do [current habit], I will also do [new habit]."

Look at these real-life examples of women I work with and how they applied habit stacking to their lives:

- "I wanted to start reading my Bible every day, and I love my morning coffee, so now I read my Bible while I drink my morning coffee."

- "I wanted to begin my mornings with prayer, so when the alarm goes off, I pray before I get out of bed."
- "I wanted to start prep-cooking for the week. I really enjoy listening to podcasts and audiobooks, so I put them on while I cook."
- "My friend and I used to always go out to eat. We wanted to get healthier, so we started working out together and praying for each other instead."
- "I love sitting outside and reading books, but God was telling me I needed to start working out. He showed me that I could enjoy the outdoors by walking and listening to my books on audio. This has been a double win!"
- "The only time I have to work out is in the morning after I drop my kids off at school. So I found a group fitness class that's on the way home at that time. Knowing that I'm going to work out after I drop them off has helped me make my workouts a habit."
- "I've wanted to memorize scriptures, so I put them on my mirror and go over them while I brush my teeth."
- "I wanted to start journaling, so I put my journal on my nightstand. When I get in bed, I tuck myself in with a bit of writing and gratitude."
- "I needed to drink more water, so in addition to drinking the water in my bottle throughout the day, I have a glass with every meal."
- "I wanted to work on accepting my body and finding confidence in who I am in Christ, so I meditate on scriptures when I get dressed for the day."
- "I wanted to focus on getting rid of stress, so I started practicing belly breathing while I watch my favorite show at the end of the day."
- "I wanted to spend time in worship, so I started listening to Christian music when I drive."

Out of the three tools and the many examples, I hope one of them encourages you to activate your faith by trying it.

> Therefore, preparing your minds for action, and being sober-minded, set your hope fully on the grace that will be brought to you at the revelation of Jesus Christ. (1 Peter 1:13 ESV)

Fit God's Way Power-Up Plan

Power-Up Points

- Activating your faith requires believing in what you do not see.
- Overcome your area of struggle with the Activate-Your-Faith Success Equation = Seek God + Surrender it daily to God + Show up in the Spirit.
- It doesn't matter how long you've been where you are or how impossible your goals seem—God wants you to get up in your inner man and live for Him!
- Get into action with the five-second rule by winning the moment in front of you and/or by learning habit stacking.

Promises

"And whatever you ask in prayer, you will receive, if you have faith." (Matthew 21:22 ESV)

So faith comes from hearing, and hearing through the word of Christ. (Romans 10:17 ESV)

"For assuredly, I say to you, whoever says to this mountain, 'Be removed and be cast into the sea,' and does not doubt in his

heart, but believes that those things he says will be done, he will
have whatever he says."
(Mark 11:23 NKJV)

Prayer

Dear God,
I'm believing, without doubting, that this mountain of not being
healthy will be removed according to Your Word (Mark 11:23).
I am asking in faith to receive this blessing (Matthew 21:22).
Father, I have really struggled in the natural, in my flesh, but in
You, through the power of the Holy Spirit working in me, I can
quickly turn my doubts, fears, and excuses into action. My faith
is being built to a whole new level by hearing your Word
(Romans 10:17). When I'm tempted to do things I know will
lead me away from the healthy and whole life You died to give
me, bring to mind the man at the healing pool in Bethesda, and
help me to get up in my spirit (John 5:5–6). I have been settling
for less than Your best for way too long. I'm activating my faith
by seeking You, surrendering this to You, and showing up in
Your Spirit! May You be glorified through my health success. In
Jesus's name, amen.

Power-Up Challenge

Get Fit God's Way with the Daily 7 Ws

(Print weekly template at www.fitgodsway.com)

Word: Read your Bible and pray.
Worth: Practice placing your worth in Christ to find
confidence, strength, and grace.
Whole, God-Made Food: Choose whole, God-made food over
man-made, processed foods. Focus on quality ingredients

versus obsessing over quantities. Pray before meals.

Water: Divide your weight in half and drink a minimum of that many ounces per day. Add seven to ten ounces of fluid every ten to twenty minutes during exercise.

Work Out: Move and strengthen your body five to six days a week. In addition, take walks outdoors to spend time in God's creation and mini-movement breaks throughout the day to increase your non-exercise activity calorie burn.

Worship: Listen to Christian music, sing, dance, and praise God.

Wake/Sleep: Establish a wake/sleep cycle and a morning/evening routine to put yourself to bed in the peace of God and wake up in His power.

HABIT 4:

Choose Fit Thoughts

How to Choose Fit Thoughts

"The Spirit of truth, whom the world cannot receive, because it nether sees Him nor knows Him; but you know Him, for He dwells with you and will be with you."

John 14:17 NKJV

I read everything I can about fitness, mindsets, and wholeness, so I have to share some astounding statistics with you.

In an interview to discuss her book *Get Out of Your Head: Stopping the Spiral of Toxic Thoughts,* author Jennie Allen said:

> We have anywhere from nine thousand to sixty thousand thoughts in a day. Of those thoughts, 85 percent, for most humans, are negative. And about 95 percent of our thoughts are repetitive from the day before. So that means that we're thinking the same negative thoughts over and over and over again.[1]

Those statistics seemed too awful to be true, but this struggle with negative thoughts is what I help women overcome daily. My email is flooded with messages from people who are desperate to get fit. As I read their words, I see repeatedly that their workouts or what they're eating isn't what's preventing their success—it's the way they think about fitness and themselves that is keeping them from reaching their fitness goals.

I bet the devil loves hearing God's daughters speaking so hatefully about and to themselves, but this should not be the case. You're not alone if negativity fills your mind—but dear sister, you don't have to keep putting up with it anymore.

Consider the things you say to and about yourself. That little voice that talks to you all day long can either be your best friend or your worst enemy. How many times today have you criticized, judged, berated, or belittled yourself? Now think about how this is affecting your motivation, your confidence, and your ability to boldly go after your goals. Is it helping you or hurting you?

Imagine sitting across a table from your best friend at lunch and talking to her the way you talk to yourself. Would she get up and leave? Would she be hurt and offended? We don't realize how much power is in our words. The Bible tells us:

> Death and life are in the power of the tongue, and those who
> love it and indulge it will eat its fruit and bear the consequences
> of their words. (Proverbs 18:21 AMP)

This scripture illustrates how important fit thinking is. Our words are shaping our lives. Consider how much power your inner voice has and what the consequences of listening to it are. Did you know that all day long, you are either talking yourself into or out of your goals? You're telling yourself, "Yes, I can!" or "No, I can't!" Tune in to your inner voice and pay attention. Listen to it; what do you hear it saying? Is it cheering you on, or is it tearing you down? If it is tearing you down, it is important to challenge it and address it.

Meet Hannah

My beautiful client Hannah had been trying to get fit and feel comfortable in her skin all her life. She said there wasn't a moment she could recall when she felt good about herself. After working with Hannah for a few weeks, I asked her how things were progressing, and she confided that she didn't believe she could ever reach her fitness goals. You should have seen the look on her face when I said, "Hannah, you're right. You can't, because you can't rise above any limit you've set for yourself."

The Bible tells us, "For as [a man] thinks in his heart, so is he" (Proverbs 23:7 NKJV). Hannah and I worked to uncover the source of her negative thoughts about herself. Through time and prayer, here's what we found:

Hannah grew up struggling with her weight. She shared a story about how she was asked to go to prom in high school. When she went shopping for a dress with her mom, she overheard her mother tell the dressing room attendant, "She's got a weight problem, like everyone in our family. I hope she picks something black." Hannah's heart sank. She said she could still picture herself looking in the dressing-room mirror and thinking, *I have a weight problem?* Her mom never knew that she had overheard her. Hannah told her mom she had decided she didn't want to go to the dance, and they left the mall.

Hannah let her mom's words that day form her view of herself. This mindset kept her trapped in a negative cycle of gaining and losing weight for the next two decades because Hannah still believed in her heart that no matter what she did, she would always be overweight.

In my research to uncover why women have negative inner conversations and why they're so hard on themselves, I read a book called *Mindset* by Carol Dweck. Carol wrote about the two types of mindsets: growth and fixed. As you read over the different characteristics of each, prayerfully ask God to reveal which one you have.

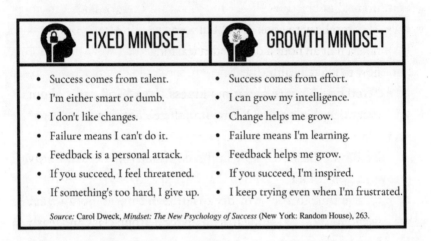

FIXED MINDSET	GROWTH MINDSET
• Success comes from talent.	• Success comes from effort.
• I'm either smart or dumb.	• I can grow my intelligence.
• I don't like changes.	• Change helps me grow.
• Failure means I can't do it.	• Failure means I'm learning.
• Feedback is a personal attack.	• Feedback helps me grow.
• If you succeed, I feel threatened.	• If you succeed, I'm inspired.
• If something's too hard, I give up.	• I keep trying even when I'm frustrated.

Source: Carol Dweck, *Mindset: The New Psychology of Success* (New York: Random House), 263.

In Fit God's Way terms, a growth mindset is a is a made-for-more mindset, and a fixed mindset is a less-than mindset. Dweck's book shows how your view of yourself can determine everything. If you believe you can't change—the fixed mindset—you will want to prove yourself correct over and over rather than learning from your mistakes. If you've ever found yourself recreating the results you don't want, this could be why. Characteristics of a fixed (less-than) mindset tend to be to be based in fear of failure and rejection. These are limiting mindsets—but we serve a limitless God who wants us thinking growth-oriented (made-for-more) thoughts.

How Our Thinking Affects Our Fitness

Notice the difference between a fixed (less-than) mindset and a growth (made-for-more) mindset:

- "I can't lose weight! I've tried everything." vs. "I'm going to believe that if I honor God with my choices, He will help me become the healthiest version of myself."

- "I'm too old, and it's too late." vs. "It's never too late for God to do a new thing in me."

- "I'm too busy to cook." vs. "I'm going to take a half an hour a day to start learning how to make healthy meals."
- "God doesn't care about my fitness." vs. "God cares about every detail in my life. With Him, there's nothing I can't do!"
- "I've never been considered pretty, and it makes me feel invisible." vs. "I am fearfully and wonderfully made. God only made one of me."
- "I don't go to the gym because I don't know how to lift weights." vs. "I'm going to sign up for a group class and learn how to lift weights."
- "I was born with bad genetics, so it doesn't matter what I eat or if I work out." vs. "I know that every meal and every workout is a step closer to my goal. God honors my faithfulness."

Learn the Habit of Fit Thoughts with the 3 Cs

"But when he, the Spirit of truth, comes, he will guide you into all the truth. He will not speak on his own; he will speak only what he hears, and he will tell you what is yet to come." (John 16:13 NIV)

Everything starts with your thoughts, so they have the power to make or break your Fit God's Way goals. Did you know the voice you listen to the most is your own? For this reason, it's vital to continually speak God's truth over yourself. Watch out for thoughts that are negative, sabotaging, based in other people's opinions of you, or based in unresolved shame or guilt. Thinking and speaking Fit Thoughts is to think and speak godly thoughts. They line up with the Word, they lead to wholeness, and they are revealed to us through the Holy Spirit, which is also called the Spirit of Truth. These are the 3 Cs:

Take Every Thought CAPTIVE, and Make It Obedient to Christ

> For the weapons of our warfare are not carnal but mighty in God for pulling down strongholds, casting down arguments and every high thing that exalts itself against the knowledge of God, bringing every thought into captivity to the obedience of Christ...(2 Corinthians 10:4–5 NKJV)

The fact that you think a thought doesn't mean you have to own it or believe it. A quick way to check is to test it against the Word. When a thought comes into your mind, ask yourself, *Is this true of what God says about me?* If it's not, reject it. It will take practice to take your thoughts captive *each time* they pop into your mind, but it is possible with the help of the Holy Spirit. Picture your mind like a flower garden—the negative thoughts are weeds. Pluck those ugly, ungodly weeds right out of your mind and plant some godly truth there to take their place.

CAST All Your Cares on Him, for He Cares for You

> Therefore, humble yourselves under the mighty hand of God...casting all your care upon Him, for He cares for you. (1 Peter 5:6–7 NKJV)

God cares about what concerns you. It's important to give Him your cares and then trust that He's working all things for your good. Once you give Him what concerns you, don't take it back. It's not easy, but practice doing your part and trusting Him to do His.

CHOOSE to Not Be Conformed to This World, but Be Transformed by the Renewing of Your Mind

And do not be conformed to this world, but be transformed by the renewing of your mind, that you may prove what is that good and acceptable and perfect will of God. (Romans 12:2 NKJV)

Spending time in the Word will train your mind to spot lies and negativity and discern what is and what is not of God. Remember the self-talk test to choose Fit Thoughts: If you wouldn't say it to your best friend or someone you greatly love and respect, then you shouldn't say it to yourself. Becoming aware of what you're thinking about is how you confront these thoughts and cure them, so look for the theme in your self-talk and collect scriptures to pray over them.

Here is an acronym I came up to shift your mindset back to God: C.A.L.M. (Christ Alone Leads Me). The following two resources can help you quickly spot where the enemy is trying to deceive you.

Choosing to think fit thoughts is important, because our thoughts affect our health, worth, identity, body image, and our ability to accomplish the plans that God has for us.

Now thanks be to God who always leads us in triumph in Christ, and through us diffuses the fragrance of His knowledge in every place. (2 Corinthians 2:14 NKJV)

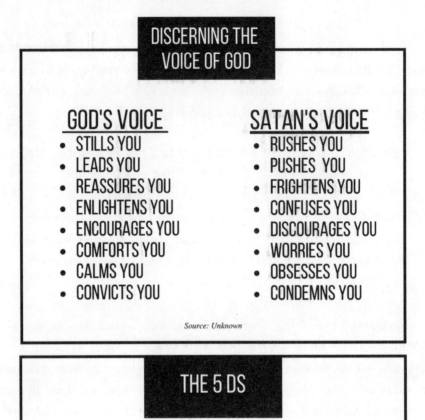

DISCERNING THE VOICE OF GOD

GOD'S VOICE
- STILLS YOU
- LEADS YOU
- REASSURES YOU
- ENLIGHTENS YOU
- ENCOURAGES YOU
- COMFORTS YOU
- CALMS YOU
- CONVICTS YOU

SATAN'S VOICE
- RUSHES YOU
- PUSHES YOU
- FRIGHTENS YOU
- CONFUSES YOU
- DISCOURAGES YOU
- WORRIES YOU
- OBSESSES YOU
- CONDEMNS YOU

Source: Unknown

THE 5 DS

Doubt	Makes you question God's Word and His goodness
Discouragement	Makes you look at your problems rather than at God
Diversion	Makes the wrong things seem attractive so that you will want them more than the right things
Defeat	Makes you feel like a failure so that you don't even try
Delay	Makes you put off doing something so that it never gets done

Source: NLT Chronological Life Application Study Bible (Carol Stream, Illinois: Tyndale, 2012).

Chapter 8

HIMpowered Worth and Identity

For we are God's masterpiece. He has created us anew in Christ Jesus, so we can do the good things he planned for us long ago.

Ephesians 2:10 NKJV

I was sitting in a circle with a group at a women's retreat. When I asked each of them to share what it means to have their identity in Christ, I was shocked to find that no one could answer me. This simple question only raised more questions. I gave them some homework for the night and asked them to come back with their answers the next day.

The homework I gave them was to watch the movie *Overcomer*. In the film, a teacher tells a young girl to read Ephesians 1 and 2

> **"Don't ever think that the sin of your past means there is no hope for your future."**
> —John Piper

and write down who God says she is. Every time you see the words "in Christ," she said, write down the words that follow; these words describe who you are in Him.

The moment I walked into the room the next morning, women started coming up to me and saying, "Thank you, you have no idea how that movie has changed my life!" I smiled and said that God and the Kendrick brothers deserved the credit!

As we went around the circle, the joy and excitement in the group were palpable, and the answers were powerful: "I'm redeemed," "I'm chosen," "I'm blessed with every spiritual blessing," "I'm loved"—and my favorite, "I'm His masterpiece created in Christ Jesus." Did you catch the last one? You are His Masterpiece. You are a piece of the Master.

> **"We serve a God who is waiting to hear from you, and He can't wait to respond."**
> —Priscilla Shirer

All too often, after we accept Christ as our Savior, the relationship becomes one of duty: going to church, attending Bible study, and saying prayers. But this is not what God had in mind when He sent His Son, Jesus, and gave us the Holy Spirit. God created us for relationship. He wants to be your best friend, your confidence, even your fitness coach—your everything!

I titled this section "HIMpowered" because we need to make God the source of our worth and our identity. Anytime we start to place our identity in things like our career, how we look, the money we make, or anything else, pride, doubt, fear, comparison, unworthiness, and shame creep in.

Made New in Christ

Our identities have been formed from our life experiences, but these events and circumstances can separate us from our worth in Christ and cause us to feel insecure, shameful, and fearful. Sadly, an identity in anything other than Christ can make us sit on the sidelines of our lives and play small to keep ourselves safe. But in Christ, we can be made new and even renewed and refreshed in Him daily.

> Therefore, if anyone is in Christ, he is a new creation; old things have passed away; behold, all things have become new. (2 Corinthians 5:17 NKJV)

Do you struggle with unresolved guilt or shame? Do you feel insecure around other women? Do you compare yourself to others, or envy those who have what you want? As you read those words, did anything come to mind? Our habit of thinking Fit Thoughts can be strengthened or shaken by where we place our identity.

This is a hand-on-your-shoulder, let's-get-free-in-Christ kind of moment. So, friend…

- Do you know who you are in Christ?
- Do you know the gifts and power you have in Him?
- Are you relying on them?

The Word Is Our Truest Strength Training

Knowing the Word of God is our truest and greatest strength training, because we have an enemy who will do anything to keep us from knowing our worth in Christ. The devil wants our focus on what we're not, so he points out everything we do wrong. But in Christ, we have power, and we can only know this power if we arm ourselves with the Word.

Remember the same power that raised Jesus from the grave lives in you! Memorize these scriptures and refer to them as often as needed:

When you struggle with past sin
  If we confess our sins, He is faithful and just to forgive us our
  sins and to cleanse us from all unrighteousness. (1 John 1:9
  NJKV)

When you feel insecure
  For You formed my inward parts;
  You covered me in my mother's womb.
  I will praise You, for I am fearfully and wonderfully made;
  Marvelous are Your works,
  And that my soul knows very well. (Psalm 139:13–14 NKJV)

When you need to remember that God has a plan for your life
"For I know the thoughts that I think toward you," says the LORD, "thoughts of peace and not of evil, to give you a future and a hope." (Jeremiah 29:11 NKJV)

When you don't know what to do
If any of you lacks wisdom, let him ask of God, who gives to all liberally and without reproach, and it will be given to him. (James 1:5 NKJV)

When you compare yourself to others
Therefore do not cast away your confidence, which has great reward. (Hebrews 10:35 NKJV)

When you need motivation
Therefore I remind you to stir up the gift of God which is in you through the laying on of my hands. (2 Timothy 1:6 NKJV)

When you need to persevere
And let us not grow weary while doing good, for in due season we shall reap if we do not lose heart. (Galatians 6:9 NKJV)

When you need self-control
For God gave us a spirit not of fear but of power and love and self-control. (2 Timothy 1:7 NKJV)

When you're struggling with fear
"Fear not, for I am with you;
Be not dismayed, for I am your God.
I will strengthen you,
Yes, I will help you,
I will uphold you with My righteous right hand.'" (Isaiah 41:10 NKJV)

When you need to forgive yourself and get back up in grace

There is therefore now no condemnation to those who are in Christ Jesus, who do not walk according to the flesh, but according to the Spirit. (Romans 8:1 NKJV)

When you're struggling with temptation

No temptation has overtaken you except such as is common to man; but God is faithful, who will not allow you to be tempted beyond what you are able, but with the temptation will also make the way of escape, that you may be able to bear it. (1 Corinthians 10:13 NKJV)

When you need to remember God can do a new thing

"Do not remember the former things,
Nor consider the things of old.
Behold, I will do a new thing,
Now it shall spring forth;
Shall you not know it?
I will even make a road in the wilderness
And rivers in the desert." (Isaiah 43:18–19 NKJV)

When you're facing trials

My brethren, count it all joy when you fall into various trials, knowing that the testing of your faith produces patience. But let patience have its perfect work, that you may be perfect and complete, lacking nothing. (James 1:2–4 NKJV)

When you've suffered a setback

And we know that all things work together for good to those who love God, to those who are the called according to His purpose. (Romans 8:28 NKJV)

When you need to find joy in the process

[F]or the joy of the Lord is your strength. (Nehemiah 8:10 NKJV)

When you need to find balance

Be sober [well balanced and self-disciplined], be alert and cautious at all times. That enemy of yours, the devil, prowls around like a roaring lion [fiercely hungry], seeking someone to devour. (1 Peter 5:8 AMP)

When you need strength

In the day when I cried out, You answered me,
And made me bold with strength in my soul. (Psalm 138:3 NKJV)

When you're dealing with anxiety

Be anxious for nothing, but in everything by prayer and supplication, with thanksgiving, let your requests be made known to God; and the peace of God, which surpasses all understanding, will guard your hearts and minds through Christ Jesus. (Philippians 4:6–7 NKJV)

When stress is getting to you

"Come to Me, all you who labor and are heavy laden, and I will give you rest. Take My yoke upon you and learn from Me, for I am gentle and lowly in heart, and you will find rest for your souls. For My yoke is easy and My burden is light." (Matthew 11:28–30 NKJV)

When you feel alone

"Be strong and of good courage, do not fear nor be afraid of them; for the Lord your God, He is the One who goes with you. He will not leave you nor forsake you." (Deuteronomy 31:6 NKJV)

<u>When you feel hopeless</u>

Now may the God of hope fill you with all joy and peace in believing, that you may abound in hope by the power of the Holy Spirit. (Romans 15:13 NKJV)

<u>When you need peace</u>

"These things I have spoken to you, that in Me you may have peace. In the world you will have tribulation; but be of good cheer, I have overcome the world." (John 16:33 NKJV)

These scriptures are just a sample of how knowing the Word of God and placing your identity in Him will HIMpower your journey toward fitness and wholeness. Hold onto them and refer to them whenever you need them.

Chapter 9

The Body-Confidence Cure: See His Perfection in Your Reflection

Your hands have made me and fashioned me.

Psalm 119:73 NKJV

The struggle to feel confident in our skin is a very real battle that we have to fight with the Word. I recently had an experience that painfully reminded me of how the enemy uses our body image to shatter our confidence.

The knock on the door shook me back to reality as the sales attendant asked, "So, how do those jeans fit?" I couldn't wrap my head around the way they looked. I had tried on over ten pairs, and nothing looked good—nothing fit. With every pair, old insecurities began to surface about my body. I blurted out, "I have to go. I'm sorry!"

As I threw my clothes on to get out of the store, I reasoned with myself that maybe it was the mirror, or the lighting, or jeans were cut differently this season—but nothing helped. I thought I was past this issue with myself. I got in my car and promised not to beat myself up—or worse, cry.

As I got in the car, my phone rang. It was a girl named Maddi, whom I had been working with, and she was very upset. She asked me, "How do I overcome my painful insecurities about how I look?" My heart sank for her. I stopped thinking about the pain of my failed shopping trip and switched gears to tell her the very thing I should've been saying to myself:

"You are not the parts and pieces people try to reduce you to. You are a whole, masterful work of Christ. God designed you, you are the work of His hands, and He doesn't make mistakes." I shared with her what the Bible had to say about body image: "But now, O Lord, you are our Father; we are the clay, and you are our potter; we are all the work of your hand." (Isaiah 64:8 ESV)

I shared with her that her value isn't external, and that God looks at her heart.

> But the Lord said to Samuel, "Do not look at his appearance or at his physical stature, because I have refused him. For the Lord does not see as man sees; for man looks at the outward appearance, but the Lord looks at the heart." (1 Samuel 16:7 NKJV)

I told her the cure for feeling insecure is this: body confidence comes from seeing His perfection in your reflection. I explained to her that she is made in the image of God. "So God created man in His own image; in the image of God He created him; male and female He created them." (Genesis 1:27 NKJV)

After a few moments, she said she felt better. I told her I'd text her those scriptures and that she should write them out and tape them to her mirror. When we got off the phone, I sat in the parking lot and felt overcome with conviction. *Why hadn't I told myself the same thing?*

Our Body Image Can Shake the Foundation of Our Fit Thoughts

Why does this happen? Why do we have to be tested over and over again? Maybe your test isn't jeans; maybe it's what people say about you or how you feel when you see yourself in pictures. But whatever makes you start to turn inward and not like the way you look is straight from the enemy. He wants your focus on what you don't like about yourself so he can stop God's plans for you. Learning to recognize that these moments are opportunities to speak God's truth over yourself will help you overcome them and make you unstoppable!

Did you know that 97 percent of women are unhappy with their appearance?[1] This statistic is sad, because it shows we're not embracing how God uniquely designed each of us. Maybe today you're chasing perfection and believe that if you can work hard enough to reach your goal weight, you'll finally feel good about yourself. Or perhaps, you've completely let yourself go and tell yourself you don't care. But I bet on either end of these extremes, there's an ache in the heart that says, "I know I'm more than this!" And friend, you are!

Have you ever wondered who or what created how you see yourself? We need to pinpoint this and align it with the Word.

Meet Karen, the perfectionist.

She was desperate to be a size 8. Growing up, she had been bullied about her weight, and the pain from that was still affecting her. She thought if she could just get skinny, she could prove everyone wrong and finally feel good about herself. Karen tried every diet, but with each attempt, her dream felt further away. She once showed me a picture on her phone of her vision board. It was covered with images of extremely fit and perfectly photoshopped women. Karen believed that the way she looked was the problem, but the true problem was how she saw herself.

We traced her motivation to pursue perfection back to something her family had said: they always referred to her as the "ugly duckling." Karen had taken that nickname and the bullying she experienced and turned them into a mission to be perfect. But after giving her the tools to place her identity securely in Christ and forgive her family and those who bullied her, she was able to embrace the individual beauty God had given her and get free from perfectionism.

Meet Susan, who tried to find comfort in not caring.

She was another extreme. At first glance, she seemed confident, but as she opened up, she shared she had given up on herself. Susan said getting older made her feel invisible, so she ate for comfort and had begun to isolate herself. At one appointment, I asked her, "Is there any part of you, even the slightest tinge in your soul, that really doesn't want to give up on yourself and knows you are more than this?" Susan grabbed my hand and said, "I really do, but I feel so old...like it doesn't matter anymore." Susan needed to be reminded that it wasn't too late, she wasn't too old, and God still had work for her to do.

Meet Christy, who kept talking herself out of her dreams.

Christy came to me because she wanted more godly confidence. She explained that she had a dream, but she kept talking herself out of it. "I'm nothing special, I'm just a mom and a wife, so no one will take me seriously," she said. When I asked her to explain, she shared that she had always wanted to be a fitness instructor, but she felt like she didn't look the part; that's why she referred to herself as "just a mom and a wife." Christy needed to break free from the limiting vision she had of herself, and she needed to know that God had placed that dream of being a fitness instructor in her heart for a reason. She now works as a part-time fitness instructor and says she can't imagine her life without the pure joy of encouraging women to live healthy lifestyles.

> "Your eyes are windows into your body. If you open your eyes wide in wonder and belief, your body fills up with light."
> —Matthew 6:22 MSG

There is no peace in living with a view of yourself that isn't based in the truth of who God says you are.

Try this exercise: Look at your child or a little one in your life who is very special to you. Think about how much you love that child and how you would do anything for him or her. Now, take all of those emotions and let this wash over you—this is how God looks at you. You are precious to Him. You are His daughter.

Seeing yourself through God's eyes without any need for identity based in what you look like—as a woman He created for His purposes, worthy and loved—brings your self-view back to its rightful place.

Whether you find yourself chasing perfection, settling for less, or even giving up on yourself, God has plans for you. If you're willing to see yourself through His eyes, you can find complete freedom and confidence.

Here's how:

1. Pinpoint who or what is creating the negative way you see yourself, and give God full control over your self-view.

2. Catch and replace the things you say about how you look—and never, ever say another bad thing about yourself again.

3. See yourself through the lens of the Word, and learn key scriptures to pray over yourself, like the ones I shared with Maddi:

- You are altogether beautiful, my darling; there is no flaw in you. (Song of Solomon 4:7 NIV)
- But now, O Lord, you are our Father; we are the clay, and you are our potter; we are all the work of your hand. (Isaiah 64:8 ESV)
- So God created man in His own image; in the image of God He created him; male and female He created them. (Genesis 1:27 NKJV)
- But the Lord said to Samuel, "Do not look at his appearance or at his physical stature, because I have refused him. For the Lord does not see as man sees; for man looks at the outward appearance, but the Lord looks at the heart." (1 Samuel 16:7 NKJV)
- Your beauty should not come from outward adornment, such as elaborate hairstyles and the wearing of gold jewelry or fine clothes. Rather, it should be that of your inner self, the unfading beauty of a gentle and quiet spirit, which is of great worth in God's sight. (1 Peter 3:3–4 NIV)

- Charm is deceptive, and beauty is fleeting; but a woman who fears the LORD is to be praised. (Proverbs 31:30 NIV)

4. Note the things, people, and places, that fuel your insecurity, and shower them with prayer.

5. Remember at all times Jesus is the cure for feeling insecure. In these moments, just say His name aloud.

Top Five Most Common Body-Image Triggers and a Go-To Power Thought to Beat Them

1. **The scale.** Numbers only have the power you give them.
2. **Social media.** Don't follow anyone who isn't following God. Body-part photos cause body-part idolatry; flee from them!
3. **Not liking how you look.** Do the very best you can with all God has given you and leave the rest to Him. Trade criticism for compassion.
4. **What other people say about your body.** Their opinion is not God's truth and therefore shouldn't be yours, either.
5. **Trying to look like you did in the past.** You can't be who you were, but you can be your best you today.

Chapter 10

Guard Your Heart

Guard your heart above all else, for it determines the course
of your life.

Proverbs 4:23 NLT

Guarding our hearts is a key part of developing the habit of thinking
Fit Thoughts. In this verse, Solomon is telling us our hearts affect who
we are, how we feel, and what we do. Guarding our hearts doesn't mean
we build physical walls around it; it means we protect it from worldly influ-
ences and keep it set on pleasing God. Sometimes what we need to guard
ourselves from is obvious, but sometimes it isn't. I once had a snake scare
that taught me a very important lesson about this.

On a cool, sunny Arizona day, I grabbed my laptop and an iced tea and
headed outside to make myself comfortable on a chaise lounge to write. I
was so excited. This day was going to be special! I was beginning a new
book, and I was praising God for the beautiful blue skies, the trees rustling
in the breeze, and the words that filled my heart. I couldn't wait to get
started. But as I sat down, something terrifying happened: I noticed a snake
out of the corner of my right eye. I was shocked. Upon closer inspection, I
saw the tell-tale rattle and froze in fear. It was a rattlesnake.

My husband was home, so I stood on the lounge chair and texted him, "911 help me!" As he flung open the door, I closed my eyes and prayed. I couldn't watch him get rid of the snake. I was so scared.

When the snake was gone, I could feel the adrenaline pumping through my body. I was shaking and thanking God that I hadn't been bitten. In just moments, God revealed a powerful message through this. I felt Him say, "I made this obvious. The devil isn't always so obvious, but he is just like that snake—sneaking around, trying to destroy you and kill my plan for you. Never forget that!"

That day, God made it clear that the devil didn't want me writing this book, but it isn't always this obvious. It's usually more subtle, and it's often found in the mundane aspects of our day-to-day lives.

> "God uses broken things. It takes broken soil to produce a crop, broken clouds to give rain, broken grain to give bread, broken bread to give strength. It is the broken alabaster box that gives forth perfume. It is Peter, weeping bitterly, who returns to greater power than ever."
>
> —Vance Havner

"Behold I give you the authority to trample on serpents and scorpions, and over all the power of the enemy, and nothing shall by any means hurt you." (Luke 10:19 NKJV)

Where is God telling you to guard your heart?

Have you ever noticed how everything in your day can be going along fine, and then something happens? It instantly makes you turn inward; makes you feel small, prideful, and jealous; tempts you to gossip, covet, or compare. We need to acknowledge it in order to guard our hearts and take away its power by giving it to God.

For freedom Christ has set us free; stand firm therefore, and do not submit again to a yoke of bondage. (Galatians 5:1 ESV)

What We Give Power to Has Power over Us

Recognizing that we can't give anything more power than we give to Jesus is a great way to immediately do a gut check. Here's a real-life example: the next time you're scrolling through your Instagram feed and see images of someone who just reached their fitness goal or launched the business you know God is calling you to start, don't let it make you feel small or insecure. Turn to God immediately and ask Him to show you how to live free, guard your heart, and live your best life. We often give our power away to things that drain the life out of our purpose and break us down. When we guard our hearts, there's a happy ending to our story because God takes the things that have broken our hearts, our confidence, and our trust, and He builds something beautiful out of them.

> **"Watch your thoughts, they become words. Watch your words, they become actions. Watch your actions, they become habits. Watch your habits, they become character. Watch your character, it becomes your destiny."**
> —Frank Outlaw

Fit God's Way Power-Up Plan

Power-Up Points

- The enemy wants to steal our health, and he does it by attacking our worth, identity, body image, and insecurities.
- In order to confront the thoughts that steal away our health and wholeness, we need to follow the 3 Cs: Captive, Cast, Choose.
- The Body-Confidence Cure is seeing His perfection in your reflection. Jesus is the cure for what makes us insecure.
- What we give our power to has power over us, so we must guard our hearts.

Promises

For You formed my inward parts;
You covered me in my mother's womb.
I will praise You, for I am fearfully and wonderfully made;
Marvelous are Your works,
And that my soul knows very well.
My frame was not hidden from You,
When I was made in secret,
And skillfully wrought in the lowest parts of the earth.
Your eyes saw my substance, being yet unformed.
And in Your book they all were written.
The days fashioned for me,
When as yet there were none of them.
(Psalm 139:13–16 NKJV)

Let the words of my mouth
and the meditation of my heart
Be acceptable in Your sight,
O Lord, my strength and my Redeemer.
(Psalm 19:14 NKJV)

Be anxious for nothing, but in everything by prayer and supplication, with thanksgiving, let your requests be made known to God; and the peace of God, which surpasses all understanding, will guard your hearts and minds through Christ Jesus. Finally, brethren, whatever things are true, whatever things are noble, whatever things are just, whatever things are pure, whatever things are lovely, whatever things are of good report, if there is any virtue and if there is anything praiseworthy—meditate on these things. (Philippians 4:6–8 NKJV)

The God of our Lord Jesus Christ, the Father of glory, may give to you the spirit of wisdom and revelation in the knowledge of Him, the eyes of your understanding being enlightened; that you may know what is the hope of His calling, what are the riches of the glory of His inheritance in the saints, and what is the exceeding greatness of His power toward us who believe, according to the working of His mighty power. (Ephesians 1:17–19 NKJV)

Prayer

Dear God,

I bring my insecurities to You and lay them at Your feet. I surrender my reputation, my body image, and my need for approval to You. I want to know the hope of Your calling and the exceeding greatness of Your power (Ephesians 1:18–19). You know the things that break me down and make me feel less-than. In these weak moments, please have mercy on me and reveal to me, through the Holy Spirit, that these are traps from the enemy. I want to turn from them and praise You, for I am fearfully and wonderfully made (Psalm 139:14). My thoughts about myself rob me of my peace, but Your Word says, "Be anxious for nothing, but in everything by prayer and supplication, with thanksgiving, let your requests be made known to God; and the peace of God, which surpasses all understanding, will guard your hearts and minds through Christ" (Philippians 4:6–8). Father, guard my heart from the things the enemy uses against me. Keep me as the apple of Your eye; hide me under the shadow of Your wings (Psalm 17:8). You are my confidence and security. When I see myself through Your eyes, I can walk in Your power and be free to be who You made me to be. In Jesus's name, amen.

Power-Up Challenge

Get Fit God's Way with the Daily 7 Ws

(Print weekly template at www.fitgodsway.com)

Word: Read your Bible and pray.

Worth: Practice placing your worth in Christ to find confidence, strength, and grace.

Whole, God-Made Food: Choose whole, God-made food over man-made, processed foods. Focus on quality ingredients versus obsessing over quantities. Pray before meals.

Water: Divide your weight in half and drink a minimum of that many ounces per day. Add seven to ten ounces of fluid every ten to twenty minutes during exercise.

Work Out: Move and strengthen your body five to six days a week. In addition, take walks outdoors to spend time in God's creation and mini-movement breaks throughout the day to increase your non-exercise activity calorie burn.

Worship: Listen to Christian music, sing, dance, and praise God.

Wake/Sleep: Establish a wake/sleep cycle and a morning/evening routine to put yourself to bed in the peace of God and wake up in His power.

HABIT 5:

Eat to Fuel Your Temple

Intentionally Choosing
God-Made Foods

"And I will pray the Father, and He will give you another Helper, that He may abide with you forever."

John 14:16 NKJV

In our fast-paced world, we often eat on autopilot, and our health is suffering as a result. We tend to choose convenience over nourishing our bodies and gravitate toward mindless eating rather than eating with intention. It's common to pour sugary cereal in a bowl before running out the door in the morning, or tell yourself, "Today is awful, so I deserve a treat," or maybe even grab your favorite fast food and emotionally numb yourself after a long day at work. These behaviors seem harmless, but they are shaping our habits and affecting our health.

Learning the habit of Intentional eating will help you carefully consider what you eat and why you eat it. It will prepare your mind for food, invite God to the table, and help you practice self-control.

Eating with intention through the power of the Holy Spirit is how we own our part in our health journey. It's how we stop the sin of gluttony, the chaos of dieting, and the deception that a protein bar from a convenience store is somehow healthier than an apple and raw nuts.

If you struggle with food, it's important to understand that there is a spiritual battle going on—and spiritual battles cannot be solved with worldly weapons.

I dieted for years. I'd lose weight and then gain it all back. I think I did what many of us do when we diet: I rode what I call the "shame train" of self-sabotage (overeating) and self-loathing (beating myself up for overeating). This cycle was fueled by the fitness industry. I would work so hard to lose weight for a shoot or a fitness show—but once I did, I had a list of foods I couldn't wait to indulge in. I felt desperate to get off that rollercoaster—until one day at church, God set me free.

This Sunday service felt different. As the worship music played, tears streamed down my face. As I cried out to God, I could feel the presence of the Holy Spirit. I couldn't take feeling this way anymore. I needed a break-through. I hadn't slept well the night before; I had woken up many times, upset with myself about what I had eaten that day. My battle to lose weight and get my eating under control was a constant dialogue in my thoughts.

We were studying Revelation, so I opened my Bible to Revelation 3:20 and was overcome by the answer before my eyes:

"Here I am, I stand at the door and knock, if anyone answers I will come in and eat with them and they with me." (NIV)

That day in church, I had a come-to-Jesus moment with eating. Reading those words changed my life: I had a revelation that Jesus wanted to eat with me. He was there to help me repair my relationship with food. He showed me that I needed to look to Him and not a diet for victory. He showed me that food, dieting, and all the guilt from whether I ate perfectly or not was an idol. He showed me that inviting Him to the table meant I told Him about my emotions rather than eating them, and if He was sitting at my table, I wouldn't be on my phone while mindlessly eating. I would be prayerful, and I would actually enjoy the food before me. He made me see that eating was something to do from a grateful heart, not a gluttonous one. God made it clear that my issue with food was a battle of my flesh against my spirit, and He was there to help me.

Here is why we must shift from mindless to intentional eating. The Bible tells us we will reap what we sow.

> Do not be deceived: God is not mocked, for whatever one sows, that will he also reap. (Galatians 6:7 NKJV)

Consider the example of the farmer here. What are you sowing (through your eating), and what are you reaping (in your health)?

This is about more than the poor-quality foods or the quantity of food you eat; this is also about how we feel about ourselves after we eat. Think about how you feel when you lose self-control and the guilt that follows. Those emotions harm your emotional and physical health. I believe dieting has caused a dis-ease relationship with food, and the dis-ease from the food we eat and the toll it takes on us are a known cause of actual disease—i.e., illness.

Did you know that emotional stress is a major contributing factor to the six leading causes of death in the United States? Cancer, coronary heart disease, accidental injuries, respiratory disorders, cirrhosis of the liver, and suicide can often be traced back to this root. Likewise, the U.S. Centers for Disease Control and Prevention estimate that stress accounts for about 75 percent of all doctor visits.[1]

Many of us eat to relieve stress, to numb emotional pain, to cope with challenging circumstances, and even to reward ourselves for accomplishments. The foods we choose are often unhealthy, so the damage is threefold—physical, emotional, and spiritual—because gluttony is a sin.

The following tool will teach you how to eat with intention and give you a simple plan you can live by to forever end mindless eating, stress-driven eating, gluttony, and the seemingly never-ending cycle of dieting failure. This is a journey to be taken meal by meal, one day at a time, so remember to replace food guilt with God's grace, and do your very best to glorify God in your body.

Learn Intentional Eating with the 7 Ps

The 7 Ps provide the daily structure to adopt the habit of intentional eating. They teach you a godly mindset toward food, because it isn't the food plan or the workout you follow that will get you fit—it's your mindset. A mind set on Christ is how you will win this battle. Have you ever considered the thoughts you think right before you eat? All too often we stand up while we eat, mindlessly snack, scroll through social media on our phones, or rush through our food. But God wants us to come before Him first, invite Him to the table, thank Him for our meal, and use the authority we have in the Holy Spirit to win these battles. Depending upon the Bible translation you are reading, the Holy Spirit is referred to as the Comforter, Advocate, Helper, or Counselor. We have this powerful gift living inside of us to guide us and give us self-control. No diet can give you the spirit of self-control; only God can do that.

> "No diet can give you the Spirit of self-control. Only God can do that."

The 7 Ps

1. PAUSE
2. PRAY
3. PREPARE
4. PORTION
5. PRACTICE
6. PLAN
7. PERSIST

- **Pause** before you decide to eat, and ask yourself if you're really hungry or if you're just feeding your emotions, boredom, or stress. This will stop impulsive eating and eating while on autopilot. Pausing readies your mind to eat with thanksgiving and self-control and gives you peace about your choices.

- **Pray** before meals. Thank God for the meal before you. Invite Him to the table. Ask God to help you eat the right foods in the right amounts and for the discipline to take care of your body (His temple). Pray to surrender your appetite to Him daily and remind yourself to do so by using my acronym S.A.F.E. (Surrender Appetite Faithfully Every Day), based on Revelation 3:20.

- **Prepare** food ahead of time and learn how to prep your meals. Batching meals is a great way to always have something healthy on hand. Pick a day of the week to shop and cook. Collect favorite recipes and learn healthy ways to make all your unhealthy favorites. Prep and cook meat, chop veggies and fruit, and cook sweet potatoes and whole grains. Make it fun "me time" by cranking up your favorite Christian playlist or podcast in the background. Get good-quality storage containers in many sizes. Once the food is cooked, put it in your airtight containers; this will help it last up to four days.

- **Portion** each meal. For one week, challenge yourself to measure everything to learn what proper food portions look like. Be mindful of the amount of food you're eating, and remember—small changes in your portion sizes equal big results over time. Eat from smaller plates and bowls. If you want to indulge in a treat, serve yourself a portion on a plate and then put the rest away. Refrain from eating out of containers, bags, boxes, or pans. "Give me just enough to satisfy my needs" (Proverbs 30:8 NLT).

- **Practice** being mindful, eating slowly and without distraction. Turn off the TV and your phone. Take the time to enjoy your food. Take smaller bites and chew them ten to twenty times apiece. Try setting your fork down between bites and thinking of food as fuel and nourishment rather than comfort or reward. Listen to your body's natural cues of hunger and fullness and eat until you're about full, not totally full. Also, practice having treats with your kids and on date nights—but don't allow one indulgence to turn into a weekend off your plan (and then a week, and then a month). Get right back on track. Remember this rule: No back-to-back eating of C.R.A.P. (C = Cooking oils that are hydrogenated, R = Refined sugars, A = Artificial sweeteners and colors, P = Processed [man-made] foods.)

- **Plan** ahead. Make healthy meals as often as you can, and always have healthy snacks on hand. Don't wait until you're hungry to find food. (I know I rarely make good choices when I am starving.) When you're going to a party or a restaurant, set a godly intention to enjoy what you're going to have, and be satisfied with that. More is not better. Anytime you hear yourself thinking *Just one more bite*, that's a cue that you're sliding into gluttony.

- **Persist** and do not give up after a bad day. Recognize that this is not a perfect journey, and we are not perfect—only Jesus is perfect. Repairing our relationship with food is a continual learning process that takes time. Acknowledge that you have power over food; food does not have power over you. Remember that you are always one God-made, healthy meal away from being back on track—so make the next meal a whole, God-made one!

Repairing Our Relationship with Food

Have you ever noticed we tend to choose either oblivion or obsession with certain topics?

I think that sweet spot in the middle, called balance, is right where Jesus wants us to live. Being obsessed with what we eat, how much we weigh, or what we look like is not only disordered—it's idolatry. Have you ever wondered what causes an unhealthy relationship with food and where the obsessive or overindulging behaviors start? In a word: dieting! Dieting won't fix your issues; it creates them. Sadly, many of us have been on diets only to gain all the weight back and more. According to a study published in September 2020, "Diets as a method of weight loss or maintenance have also come under scrutiny because they lead to long-term weight gain instead." This is exacerbated by the relationship with food dieting creates. "Little emphasis has been made on the harmful effects of dieting, although some have linked its association with eating disorders."[2]

Meet Lisa

Lisa enjoyed cooking, and her food diary was like a spreadsheet of macros and calories—but her happiness and wholeness were a painful place of struggle. Lisa thought that if she prepped and cooked all her meals, recorded every bite she took, and ate perfectly, somehow she'd feel good about herself. But she didn't. In fact, her preoccupation with the numbers was completely stealing her joy! I understood what she was going through, because I had once made fitness and food an idol too, so I was able to help her. I taught her to seek Jesus first and surrender this to Him, and that He wanted her to have a healthy, balanced relationship with food, fitness, and her body. After a few months, Lisa said she realized how much trying to be perfect was making her miserable.

For some of us, food is a very real issue, and it's standing in the way of our health goals, our fitness success, and our wholeness as human beings. We want to get healthy, but food is a coping mechanism for a deeper issue, an ever-present thought in our minds, or we're enslaved by macronutrient splits and calorie counts. Whichever end of the spectrum you fall on, begin showering these thoughts in prayer and remember these scriptures:

Ask God to Reveal the Foods That Have Power over You

All things are lawful for me, but all things are not helpful. All things are lawful for me, but I will not be brought under the power of any. (1 Corinthians 6:12 NKJV)

What Paul is saying here is that we must allow nothing to enslave us in sinful habits. If you struggle with gluttony, which foods or drinks have control over you? Or, on the other end of the spectrum, which extreme diets have you tried, and how did they control you with rigid rules and false promises?

Enjoy Food without Guilt and Condemnation

Nothing *is* better for a man *than* that he should eat and drink, and *that* his soul should enjoy good in his labor. This also, I saw, was from the hand of God. (Ecclesiastes 2:24 NKJV)

Take note of how you think and feel when you eat. Afterward, do you feel guilty? Do your thoughts condemn you? If so, these are worldly dieting teachings and not of God. Begin to view food as a gift of nourishment that fuels your body to accomplish the work He has called you to.

Know You're Not Alone in Your Struggle

For we do not have a High Priest who cannot sympathize with our weaknesses, but was in all points tempted as we are, yet without sin. (Hebrews 4:15 NKJV)

We're not alone in our weaknesses. Jesus was not only tempted just like we are, but He overcame the temptation—and in Him, we can overcome it, too. This overcoming is found in learning to say no and in getting back on track quickly when we totally miss it. Think progress, not perfection. Don't spend any time beating yourself up when you blow it; instead, pray this scripture back to God, and He will help you.

Find Balance and Avoid Extreme, Man-Made Diets

Be well balanced (temperate, sober of mind), be vigilant and cautious at all times; for that enemy of yours, the devil, roams around like a lion roaring [in fierce hunger], seeking someone to seize upon and devour. (1 Peter 5:8 AMP)

Being sober of mind is central to intentional eating. The enemy wants you to engage in extreme behavior because he can devour you in those places. Be cautious with foods that you know you can't control yourself around, and be wary of the extremes of trying to eat perfectly.

Recognize the Spiritual Battle with Food

But put on the Lord Jesus Christ, and make no provision for the flesh, to fulfill its lusts. (Romans 13:14 NKJV)

People joke about food being a legal drug, but it's not funny. I recently saw this tweet from a rapper and actor named Fat Joe. He said, "Food is like a legal drug. You can take 50 cents and walk into the store and buy a Twinkie and get high. And it's killing people."

Have you ever wondered why eating one chip or cookie sometimes turns into devouring a whole bag? It's because the chemicals in these foods are as addictive as drugs like cocaine and morphine.[3]

Food is a place of spiritual battle. The devil tempted Jesus with food; Luke 4:1–13 tells us in the wilderness, Jesus endured the devil's temptation. He had fasted for forty days, "and the devil said to Him, 'If You are the Son of God, command this stone to become bread.'" Consider Eve and how the enemy tempted her with fruit, and how Esau sold his birthright to Jacob for a bowl of soup.

I believe the enemy takes what God made for natural use and perverts, twists, and creates an unhealthy relationship with it. Look at these examples:

- God made sex for marriage, but the enemy perverted it into pornography, lust, fornication, and infidelity.
- God gave us gifts to help us earn a living and to bless others, but the devil wants us to use our gifts for greed and personal gain.
- God gave us food to enjoy, but the devil uses it to destroy our physical, emotional, and spiritual health through disease, guilt, and gluttony.

Whoever sows to please their flesh, from the flesh will reap destruction; whoever sows to please the Spirit, from the Spirit will reap eternal life. (Galatians 6:8 NIV)

How to Take Down the Spirit of Gluttony

In all my years of going to church, I have never heard a message about gluttony. While I understand that it is uncomfortable to discuss, God has convicted me that it's important to talk about how it is affecting our health and fitness. As Christians, we have a hierarchy of sin—we're quick to judge an alcoholic, gambler, or adulterer, but we view the sin of gluttony as harmless. In reality, it's a form of idolatry.

Easton's Bible Dictionary tells us a "glutton," as first referenced in Deuteronomy 21:20, is the Hebrew word *zolel*, a word meaning "to shake out" or "to squander." It means one who is prodigal, who wastes his means through indulgence. As used in Proverbs 23:21, the word means "debaucher" or "waster of his own body."[4]

When I read that, I prayed for myself and other women who love Jesus to have a lightbulb moment. We often choose our own hierarchies of sin, don't we? We take adultery seriously while esteeming gluttony lightly—but sin is sin. And we want NO part of it! The Bible warns us that we cannot serve the god of our bellies.

> For many walk…whose end is destruction, whose god is their belly, and whose glory is in their shame—who set their mind on earthly things. (Philippians 3:18–19 NKJV)

Don't Take the Bait, Literally!

Have you ever heard someone say, "If you won't make time for your wellness, you will be forced to make time for your illness"? It hits hard here. Satan wants to steal your health, and he knows exactly where you struggle.

Intentional eating creates peace. Peace with food means nothing is off-limits—which is not exactly what you'd think you'd read here in a book about getting healthy. Our culture has taught us that we need to strictly diet and punish ourselves in order to lose weight. This is not true.

The dieting mentality is the problem, and it sounds like this: "You're good if you eat perfectly and a failure if you don't." Telling yourself, *I can't eat that* can cause deprivation deep within your soul that leads to food lust and ends in overindulging. Instead of saying, "I can't," reframe it and say, "Nothing is off-limits." I know this is a challenge, but you'll find you crave what dieting tells you is off-limits a lot less if you are allowed to eat whatever you want.

Be on the lookout for the thoughts, foods, and situations that make you want to be gluttonous—and don't take the bait. Begin to notice what causes you to engage in self-love, comfort, and control through food or tempts you to be a "waster of your own body." Note the cycle, and focus on how you feel after you've fallen for this trap. We can't just use positive talk to love ourselves into fitness; we must be intentional and rely on the Holy Spirit.

Grace Always Wins!

When you mess up (raising my hand here), find comfort in knowing that we all do. There is no need to beat yourself up. Don't waste a moment in self-loathing, because this is exactly what the enemy wants you to do. The longer he can keep you living in your head and believing you're a failure, the further he can take you from your health and wholeness. Don't give the devil a foothold here; otherwise, he'll turn one not-so-good choice into a weekend of not-so-good choices—and then a month of them could turn into a year!

Instead, when you do engage in gluttonous behavior, ask God to forgive you, and skip the guilt. He didn't create all the rigid rules about food and extremes of dieting to force your body to look a certain way—the world did. We need to retrain our brains from focusing on extremes to focusing on grace, because grace always wins.

> For the kingdom of God is not eating and drinking, but righteousness and peace and joy in the Holy Spirit. (Romans 14:17 NKJV)

Chapter 11

How to Eat God-Made Foods Mini-Course

"My people are destroyed for lack of knowledge."

Hosea 4:6 NKJV

I thought long and hard about even putting this section in the book, because Fit God's Way is NOT a diet or a worldly plan. However, we live in the world—and as your Fit Sister-in-Christ, certified fitness instructor, and specialist in fitness nutrition, I don't want you to get tricked into continually thinking there's some way to cheat or short-circuit the process. I want to educate you, hoping that if you know and understand how weight loss works, you will be empowered to take authority over your health and create lasting results.

Meet Kristi

Although Kristi read fitness blogs and googled workouts, she said she "always ended up feeling overwhelmed and confused about what to do." I remember the cool spring morning we sat down to chat at a coffee shop. Kristi had seen a post on Facebook that said, "Calorie counting is out, macro splits are in," so she wanted to try macros. I smiled and said, "Let's say a prayer and get to work!" After we prayed, she shared that her goal was to lose weight—specifically fat—and to gain some muscle mass. I asked if she had ever calculated how many calories she should be eating or if she understood the calories-in, calories-out energy balance model. She hadn't.

I explained to her that Fit God's Way does not advocate obsessively counting calories for daily life. However, God wants us to acquire knowledge, so my goal was to provide her with the same information she would receive from a trainer or nutritionist on the basic foundations of weight loss, fat loss, and gaining muscle.

We started by calculating her Basal Metabolic Rate (BMR) and her Total Daily Energy Expenditure (TDEE).

Understanding Methods of Weight Loss

BMR

If you hired a trainer or nutritionist, they would calculate your Basal Metabolic Rate (BMR), which is the amount of energy your body uses during a twenty-four-hour period for basic functions like breathing and digesting food. It doesn't include any physical activity.

Your BMR is part of the equation used to determine how many calories your body needs in a day. It is the sum of your age, weight, and height. There are other numbers in that formula, but don't get overwhelmed—just plug in the ones that apply to you. (I've included a worksheet in the Appendix for your personal use.)

The formula is:
BMR = (4.536 x weight) + (15.88 x height) − (5 x age) − 161[1]

Let's walk through this using Kristi's example. She weighs 160 pounds. She is 5'4" and 47 years old.

Kristi's BMR equation:

(4.536 x 160 pounds) + (15.88 x 64 inches) – (5 x 47) – 161

Therefore, Kristi's BMR is:

725.76 + 1,016.32 – 235 – 161 = 1,346.08

A quick word of advice: Keep it simple and use an online calculator to determine your BMR and TDEE. The goal of this exercise is to teach you how many calories you should be eating to support your fitness goals.

TDEE

Total Daily Energy Expenditure (TDEE) is an estimation of how many calories you burn each day, including physical activity. It is calculated by multiplying your BMR by 1.2 to 1.9, based on your activity level.

Think of your TDEE as adding everything you do in a normal day to your BMR calculation—your workouts, showering, walking around the office, taking out the trash, playing with your kids, walking the dog, doing laundry, etc. How do you know which number between 1.2 and 1.9 to use? Here are some examples.

- **Sedentary:** *I don't exercise.* Multiply BMR by 1.2.
- **Lightly Active:** *I lightly exercise 1 to 3 days per week.* Multiply BMR by 1.375.
- **Moderately Active:** *I exercise 3 to 5 days per week.* Multiply your BMR by 1.55.
- **Very Active:** *I'm an athlete or I exercise 6 to 7 days per week.* Multiply your BMR by 1.725.
- **Extra Active:** *I exercise every day and have a physically demanding job.* Multiply your BMR by 1.9.

Kristi was moderately active, so we multiplied her BMR of 1,346 by activity level of 1.55 to find that her TDEE was 2,086 calories.

Based on this number, if her calories are equal to her TDEE, she will maintain her current weight; if her calories are lower, she will lose weight; if they're higher, she will gain weight.

There are 3,500 calories in a pound. Therefore, in order for Kristi to lose a pound a week, she will have to burn 500 more calories each day for a week than what she takes in; this is known as a caloric deficit. She can accomplish this through what she eats and her workouts.

A Word about BMI

You might be wondering why I did not discuss body mass index, which is a tool suggesting how much you "should" weigh based on your height. While BMI is often used in medical settings, it was developed in 1832 and has limitations. For example, it doesn't take muscle mass into account—and while a pound is a pound, a pound of muscle takes up far less space than a pound of fat. Many experts say simply taking your waist measurement may be a better indicator of your health than using your BMI. (A waist measurement under 35 is considered ideal for women to avoid health issues.)

Should You Count Calories?

The goal of this section is to help you gain an understanding of how many calories you need to eat and what that looks like in food servings. If you've never done this before, it's very helpful in understanding the role food plays in reaching your fitness goals.

Here are some interesting facts about calories: They are a measure of energy. The energy balance model gives us the calories-in, calories-out equation, which yields these guidelines:

- When you eat more calories than you burn, you gain weight.
- When you burn more calories than you eat, you lose weight.
- When the calories you eat are equal to the calories you burn, you maintain your weight.

Calories do count, but they are far from the whole picture. We are not machines. While it may sound perfect on paper to "eat this number of calories to lose weight," it isn't that easy. Many other factors play a role in weight loss, including the quality of the calories you eat, the amount of muscle mass you have, your genetics, your hormones, diseases, and your body type.

All calories are not created equally. For example, an 8-ounce bag of potato chips has 1,200 calories in it. While many people assume that's one serving, it's actually eight servings. You could spend those 1,200 calories—almost the equivalent of an entire day's worth of meals—by eating the whole bag of chips, or you could do eat this:

- Breakfast: Overnight oats made with Greek yogurt, berries, and chia seeds (325 calories)
- Snack: A cup of raspberries (85 calories) and 10 almonds (70 calories) (155 calories total)
- Lunch: 4 ounces of grilled chicken breast (187 calories) on one cup of spinach (7 calories), topped with avocado slices (80 calories) and 2 tablespoons of balsamic vinaigrette (90 calories) (364 calories total)
- Dinner: 5 ounces of grilled salmon (242 calories) with a five-inch-long sweet potato (112 calories) and one cup of broccoli (31 calories) (385 calories total)

Isn't that shocking?!

God-made foods are high-quality, healthy foods.

Knowledge Is Powerful

Can we be so all-or-nothing? It seems like we either want to obsessively count every calorie and track our food and measurements, or we want to eat whatever we want, avoid measurements, and avoid the scale like the plague. But ignoring all the math doesn't work any better than obsessing over it.

What we need to do is what God instructs us to do: acquire knowledge in order to create a healthy lifestyle based on eating whole, God-made foods. It is powerful to take the time to understand what you're eating, what serving sizes are, and how to make meals and snacks that support your health and your goals.

Meet Amy

Amy thought she was eating really healthy, so she was stunned when we did the math and found out that she was eating more than 3,000 calories a day. This happened because she had never figured out what food serving sizes looked like. For example, she was eating a cup of walnuts (eight ounces) on her morning oats instead of the recommended one-ounce serving size. This difference accounted for more than 500 calories a day.

So I taught her a couple of simple tricks: buy baking pieces of walnuts instead of whole walnuts, and keep the measuring spoon in the jar where she stored them. Amy put all the tools in this section into practice and was able to get to a healthy weight in twelve weeks.

To acquire wisdom, challenge yourself to:

- Find an online BMR and TDEE calculator.
- Figure out your BMR and TDEE numbers.
- Write down the number of calories you should be eating.
- Write down everything you eat and drink in a typical day. We tend to eat the same things, so keep the nutritional information on a note on your phone, in your journal, or on one of the many apps that are available, like MyFitnessPal, Lose It, or Cronometer.

- Figure out the number of servings and calorie counts of these foods and drinks.
- Evaluate whether you are eating more or less than the serving sizes.
- Adjust your servings or food choices to be consistent with your goals.
- Practice measuring servings and counting calories until you have a solid foundation.
- To avoid number idolatry and perfectionism, switch to using the hand-portion method of figuring out serving sizes for foods, or use your general understanding of what portion sizes look like.
- Practice the 7 Ps.

We'll discuss macronutrients and their sources in more detail later, but for now, here's an easy way to determine portion sizes for proteins, carbohydrates, and fats.

Food Servings

<u>Protein:</u> 3 ounces, or the size of the palm of your hand
<u>Starchy Carbs:</u> 1/2 cup, or a rounded handful
<u>Fibrous Carbs:</u> 1 cup, or the size of your fist
<u>Good Fats:</u> 1 tsp, or the size of your index fingertip for cooking oils; 2 tbsp, or the length of your thumb from the knuckle to the tip for nut butters; 1/4 cup, or one handful for nut servings
<u>Condiments:</u> 2 tbsp, or two thumb joints to fingertips

Although the Fit God's Way of eating is to choose God-made foods over man-made, processed foods, it's important to learn all the numbers so you can look at food and know the serving sizes. We can't know what we don't learn.

Peace with food and lasting results don't come from man-made, hard-and-fast rules. So instead of obsessing about calories, learn about them, learn servings sizes of foods, eat God-made foods, and avoid foods that make you feel gluttonous.

Understanding How Common Diets Work

All diets are based on controlling your overall food consumption. Their differences lie in manipulating macros, removing foods, or counting calories.

Macro diets, like Keto and Atkins, eliminate carbohydrates. Carbs make your body hold onto more water, so the weight you initially lose on these diets is mainly water loss, not fat loss. Not eating bread, pasta, chips, oats, and potatoes means you naturally eat less.

HAND CHART FOR FOOD SERVINGS

Hand Symbols	Equivalent	Foods
	Fist 1 cup	Fibrous Carbs
	Palm 3 ounces	Protein
	Handful 1/2 cup	Starchy Carbs
	2 Handfuls 1 cup	Salad
	Thumb 1 ounce	Nut Butter Condiments
	Thumb Tip 1 teaspoon	Oils

Macros seem to take the focus off of calories, but they control calories by controlling your food intake.

Let's use Kristi's TDEE of 2,086 calories to figure out her macros. We'll use a common macro split of 40 percent carbs, 30 percent protein, and 30 percent fat. Notice that calculating macros is based on calories, and macros can be any type of food.

Carbohydrates have 4 calories per gram; protein has 4 calories per gram; fat has 9 calories per gram.

So, to achieve 40 percent carbohydrates:

2,086 calories x 0.40 carbohydrates = 834 calories divided by 4 (because there are 4 calories per grams of carbohydrates) = 208 grams of carbs

To find out how much 40 percent protein is:

2,086 calories x 0.30 protein = 626 calories divided by 4 (because there are 4 calories per grams of protein) = 156 grams of protein

Likewise, to find out what 30 percent fats looks like:
2,086 calories x 0.30 fat = 626 calories divided by 9 (because there are 9 calories per grams of fat) = 70 grams of fat

So Kristi's final macro split would be 208 grams of carbohydrates, 156 grams of protein, and 70 grams of fat per day.

Should You Count Macros?

The problem with macros is that unless you're an athlete who needs to prioritize protein or carbs for muscle building and recovery, have Type 1 diabetes and need to know how many carbs you're eating to properly dose insulin, or you're a fitness competitor who's trying to manipulate your body composition for a competition, eating this way can cause a lot of stress about the numbers and what exactly to eat. Also, research suggests that it doesn't necessarily yield better results than eating balanced meals and working out.

Counting macros may also create disordered eating or fuel an existing eating disorder. Macro dieting doesn't take into account the source of your macros; you can eat whatever you want as long as it stays within the macro split. So, by that philosophy, whether you're eating ice cream or bacon, as long as you stay in your macro split, you're fine.

Paleo and Whole 30 are very similar plans. They don't allow bread, rice, peanut butter, beans, cheese, yogurt, milk, or butter, so you naturally end up eating fewer calories while following them. Your weight loss occurs as result of food elimination.

I came across a study done at Stanford University comparing the outcomes of popular diets. The researchers put six hundred overweight adults on either a healthy low-fat diet or low-carb diet for twelve months and found they had similar results. The researchers wanted to find out why; they ran tests but couldn't make any connections. In the end, their recommendations for the best way to lose weight were focus on eating more veggies, less sugar, and more whole foods.[2]

God never intended for us to have a controlling and unhealthy relationship with food. Unless we have allergies or intolerances, all of His foods are for our enjoyment. We eat *food*, not macros or calories, so strict rules don't work in the long run. However, equipping ourselves with knowledge goes a long way in understanding what to eat and how much to eat so we can make informed choices and steward our temples well. Think about Amy and how measuring her walnuts saved her 500 calories a day! Little changes add up to big differences.

"The Lord himself goes before you and will be with you; he will never leave you nor forsake you. Do not be afraid; do not be discouraged."
—Deuteronomy 31:8 NIV

Food Intolerances and Allergies

If you're experiencing food sensitivities, it's important to pinpoint them. You may not even know that your migraine, achy joints, bloating, or runny nose is coming from the gluten, dairy, or other foods you eat. I highly recommend food-sensitivity testing to give yourself a full picture of your health.

After years of eating my favorite Greek yogurt, I started to have congestion and an itchiness in my throat. I suspected it was the dairy, so I stopped eating it for a couple weeks and the symptoms went away. When I tried to eat it again, the symptoms came back even worse. To confirm my suspicions, I had a food-sensitivity test, and it showed I had an extreme inflammatory response to dairy. Eliminating dairy from my diet eliminated my symptoms and prevented the health issues I would have had if I'd ignored my body.

> **"An intelligent heart acquires knowledge, and the ear of the wise seeks knowledge."**
> —Proverbs 18:15 ESV

Health Numbers

Before you begin a new plan of eating or exercising, schedule a routine visit with your doctor and get a blood panel done to give you a full picture of your health. Important health numbers to know are your blood pressure, resting heart rate, cholesterol, thyroid function, hormones, and blood sugar levels. If you've been unable to lose weight, getting blood work done could reveal any issues that are preventing you from reaching your goals.

A special note: Numbers are NOT your report card! Maybe you're like me and you need to ask God to heal your relationship with numbers. About ten years ago, my husband decided he was going to start weighing himself every day. So annoying, right?! He would hop on the scale every morning without a care in the world, and I would roll my eyes. All of my years of dieting failures, unwelcomed comments from people about my body, and the stress of getting weighed at doctor's appointments made me loathe the scale. I would've just about gotten a root canal before I stood on that thing.

Then one morning, I heard my husband get on the scale and say, "It's just a number!" and I felt deeply convicted.

Numbers, whether they were my weight, measurements, or my clothing size, had been an idol that I needed to lay down. That day, God used my husband to show me I wasn't free from this yet—but I needed to be.

The next morning, I decided to try it. I got on the scale every day for one week to see what would happen and how I'd feel. It felt foreign to me, and the first two days, I didn't like it at all. On day five, though, I started not to care about the number anymore. I watched my body fluctuate a bit through the week, and then all of a sudden, God showed me the scale had lost its grip over me. I didn't have to get down to my birthday suit and even take out my ponytail holder to get on the scale anymore. I just got on it, and it was just a number.

Track Your Progress: Gain Wisdom

If you struggle with the scale, taking your measurements, calculating your BMR and TDEE, or learning serving sizes, ask God to help you to gain a heart of wisdom without judgment. It's important to remember that numbers only have the power we give them. Instead of using numbers to be hard on yourself, view them as information. When you know what you're eating, how much you're eating, and all of the serving sizes, you will be equipped to make informed choices that lead you straight to your goals.

Kristi's Funny Story with a Successful Ending

As Kristi and I crunched the numbers, she leaned across the table, grabbed my arm, and said, "Kim, how long is this going to take?" I told her to picture the weight she wanted to lose and the calories she wanted to burn as if they were amounts she had to pay off on her credit card. That excess debt would need to be paid off before she would be able to reach her goal.

- Every workout was a payment.
- Every God-made meal was like writing another check.
- Every healthy choice reduced her debt even more.

Kristi ended up losing fat and even gaining some muscle. She said the credit card debt example was her turning point. Kristi thought of it every day and it pushed her, because she wanted to get out of debt and be a good steward of the body God had blessed her with.

Chapter 12

Why Eat God-Made Foods?

D oesn't it make sense that if God made our bodies, we should be eating the foods He designed us to eat?

> Then God said, "Let Us make man in Our image, according to Our likeness; let them have dominion over the fish of the sea, over the birds of the air, and over the cattle, over all the earth and over every creeping thing that creeps on the earth." So God created man in His own image…(Genesis 1:26–27 NKJV)

> "Every moving thing that lives shall be food for you. I have given you all things, even as the green herbs." (Genesis 9:3 NKJV)

We have the freedom to eat what we want—and as much as we may want God to tell us exactly what to eat, the truth is, there isn't a macro split or diet in the Bible. But we can still glean a lot of wisdom from it for our physical health as well as our spiritual, mental, and emotional health.

Have you ever wondered what Jesus ate? If you're anything like me, you love any details you can learn about Him. I did some research and found out these are the foods He most likely ate:

- Figs
- Raisins
- Dates
- Fish
- Lamb
- Honey
- Olive oil
- Olives
- Grapes
- Vinegar
- Bread
- Almonds
- Pistachios
- Walnuts
- Legumes
- Chickpeas
- Pomegranates
- Cucumbers
- Melons
- Mustard
- Mint
- Dill
- Leeks
- Onions
- Garlic

In other words, Jesus's diet consisted mostly of whole foods that God Himself made—and we can follow His example for optimum health.

Switch from Processed, Man-Made Foods to Whole, God-Made Foods

I'm asked multiple times a day:

- What diet are you on?
- What diet should I try?
- What's the best diet?

After twenty years in the fitness industry and trying just about every diet available, I learned the hard way what works—and it's not a dieting. It's eating whole, God-made foods. You may be wondering if it could really be that simple, and the answer is yes. Ask yourself this: when you decide what to eat, do you ever consider what you are putting in your body and how it came to be set in front of you? God created specific foods for our nourishment. These are the fruits and vegetables that grow from our earth, the water that feeds them, and the animals who graze upon them. These foods have been provided for our benefit and our sustenance, and by focusing our efforts on God-made foods versus man-made foods, our bodies will thrive.

> **"For he satisfies the longing soul, and the hungry soul he fills with good things."**
> —Psalm 107:9 ESV

Look at some of the top benefits of choosing God-made foods over man-made foods:

- Healthy weight
- Increased energy
- Reduced inflammation
- Lower cholesterol
- Stable blood sugar
- Balanced hormones
- Reduced cravings
- Greater mental acuity
- Better sleep
- Improved mental health and confidence

Our bodies weren't made to eat man-made, processed foods. Look at the contrast in how they affect our bodies.

Man-made, processed foods cause:

- Weight gain
- Decreased energy
- Inflammation
- High bad cholesterol

- Increased blood sugar
- Activation of fat-storing hormones
- Cravings
- Brain fog
- Disrupted sleep
- Contribute to anxiety, depression, and lower self-esteem

Man-made foods are processed foods, and they are the leading cause of obesity. Here are examples:

- White flour
- White sugar
- Trans fats
- Candy
- Crackers
- Chips
- Cereals
- Soda
- Fried food
- Pastries

Understanding what to eat can be very confusing in the world we live in. We hear contradictory opinions every day, so a simple rule to follow is this: Did God make it, and can I read (and understand) all of the ingredients in it? Ask God for wisdom, and He will give it to you.

If any of you lacks wisdom, let him ask of God, who gives to all liberally and without reproach, and it will be given to him. (James 1:5 NKJV)

You might have heard that nutritionists and fitness coaches agree that how we look is 80 percent what we eat and 20 percent working out.

Others say that food is 90 percent of the battle. But rather than getting caught up in these percentages, making this one change is the simplest way to get healthy: replace man-made, processed foods with healthy, God-made ones.

On a daily basis, I teach women to change their eating from man-made to God-made, so you are not alone if you experience any of these issues:

- Needing to retrain your taste buds because you are addicted to the artificial taste of man-made processed foods.
- Not realizing how important what you eat is to your health and weight loss.
- Choosing convenient, cheap food in large portions over choosing God's best foods in proper servings.

Meet Gina

When I was working with Gina, she really struggled with eating vegetables; she said they tasted awful. Gina was used to pouring processed cheese sauce all over her broccoli. After two weeks of getting rid of the man-made sauces, she texted me to say, "I'm shocked! I actually love the taste of tomatoes and broccoli now!"

The foods we choose to eat affect every cell in our bodies. Food is said to be the best medicine because it can prevent or fight disease. Eating foods that God made for your body is an easy way to know you're making the best choices. What's fast might seem like the effortless choice, but when it comes to man-made, processed food, what you're saving now in time and money will be something you pay for big-time in health issues down the road.

God-made food is self-regulating and actually satisfies your hunger. Think about it like this: Would you ever eat five chicken breasts or a dozen apples? Of course not—but devouring a big bag of French fries from the drive-through sure is easy!

We are blessed to be able to drive to a grocery store and purchase food to cook for our families. Can you imagine if we had to walk to get water from a well, pick our own berries, and fish for our own dinners? We need to change our perspective from wanting the ease of processed food to the privilege of being able to care for ourselves and our families. We don't *have* to; we *get* to.

Chapter 13

God-Made Carbohydrate Sources

The chart on the following page is a helpful tool you can print out and keep on your refrigerator to help you make good choices in moments of weakness.

Carbohydrates are your body's main source of energy and fiber; they help us feel full. Carbohydrates are essential for producing energy and building muscle. Even God has a recipe for bread in the Bible:

"And you, take wheat and barley, beans and lentils, millet and emmer, and put them into a single vessel and make your bread from them. During the number of days that you lie on your side, 390 days, you shall eat it." (Ezekiel 4:9 ESV)

Many people think that when they want to lose weight, they must cut all carbs from their food plan, when in reality, it's the *source* of carbs that is the issue. Carbs are similar to calories in the sense that they are not all created equally. For example, Ezekiel bread is radically different from man-made white bread. Ezekiel

GOD-MADE CARBOHYDRATE SERVINGS

Starchy Carbs: 1/2 cup or a rounded handful

Fibrous Carbs: 1 cup or the size of your fist

GOD-MADE FIBROUS CARBOHYDRATES

Vegetables: broccoli, spinach, kale, salad greens, green beans, carrots, peppers, eggplant, artichokes, onions, Brussels sprouts, celery, cauliflower, mushrooms, radishes, sprouts, and zucchini

GOD-MADE SIMPLE CARBOHYDRATES

Fruits: apples, oranges, grapes, bananas, berries, cherries, pears, plums, peaches, pineapple, and watermelon

GOD-MADE STARCHY CARBOHYDRATES

Potatoes, sweet potatoes, butternut squash, peas, beans, brown rice, wild rice, quinoa, farro, corn, lentils, chickpeas, yams, parsnips, and taro root.

Whole grains and foods made from them, such as oatmeal, whole-grain pasta, whole-grain crackers, and whole-grain breads.

- CHOOSE NON-GMO AND PESTICIDE-FREE SOURCES
- THIS IS NOT AN EXHAUSTIVE LIST OF ALL THE VEGETABLES, FRUITS, AND STARCHY CARBOHYDRATE SOURCES

bread contains complex, starchy, and fibrous carbohydrates, which are whole and unrefined. It is rich in fiber, satisfying, and healthy. Complex, God-made carbohydrates are commonly found in whole-plant foods and are high in vitamins and minerals. But man-made, processed, simple carbohydrates like white breads are full of sugar. They're the foods you can't seem to get full on, and they are very low in fiber.

Examples include:

- White-flour bread and pasta
- Packaged chips, crackers, cookies, and cereals
- Jams and jellies
- Table sugar
- Ice cream and candy
- Sodas and most fruit juices

Man-Made Carbohydrates

Man-made, processed carbohydrates are one of the main reasons Americans battle obesity. It's very easy to overconsume these foods, and what doesn't get burned up for energy gets stored as body fat. The Fit God's Way goal is to limit our intake of these foods and choose God-made sources.

Here are nine reasons to avoid them:

- They increase body fat and are the leading cause of obesity.
- They are full of empty calories—causing hunger even after a meal.
- They raise low-density lipoprotein (bad) cholesterol.
- They suppress our immune systems.
- They are full of chemicals that our bodies were not made to digest.
- They raise the risk of diabetes.
- They are addictive.
- They are linked to depression and fatigue.
- They alter our taste buds and make healthy foods less appetizing.

A Key to Choosing Carbohydrates

The goal of Fit God's Way is to give you tools that make you healthy and wise, including the glycemic index. This is a nutritional tool that rates the quality of a carbohydrate by how quickly it impacts your blood sugar. Here's how it works:

When our blood sugar is high, our body doesn't send the signal to burn fat (our energy reserve source). Instead, high blood sugar encourages fat storage.

As a point of reference, table sugar has a glycemic index of 100.

Low-glycemic carbs (GI of 55 or less): Most fruits and vegetables, beans, minimally processed grains, pasta, low-fat dairy foods, and nuts

Moderate glycemic carbs (GI 56 to 69): White and sweet potatoes, corn, white rice, couscous, breakfast cereals

High-glycemic carbs (GI of 70 or higher): White bread, rice cakes, most crackers, bagels, cakes, doughnuts, croissants, most packaged breakfast cereals[1]

A low-glycemic diet can help you control your weight by minimizing spikes in your blood sugar and insulin levels. This is particularly important if you have Type 2 diabetes or are at risk of developing it. Low-glycemic diets have also been linked to reduced risks for cancer, heart disease, and other conditions.[2]

Sugar is carefully hidden on many labels, and it doesn't have any nutritional value. While there's nothing wrong with occasionally enjoying ice cream or cookies, we need to retrain our taste buds to desire God's naturally sweet foods, such as fruit.

Here is a list of some of the different names of sugar to help you know what to look for on labels. They're pretty easy to spot, as they all tend to end in -ose:

- Syrup (such as high-fructose corn syrup)
- Caramel
- Molasses
- Fructose (natural sugar from fruits)
- Lactose (natural sugar from milk)
- Sucrose (common table sugar; made from fructose and glucose)

- Maltose (sugar made from grain)
- Glucose (natural sugar, product of photosynthesis)
- Dextrose (a form of glucose)

Registered dietitian Cassie Bjork, founder of the website Redefined Weight Loss, told Healthline for an April 2020 article that sugar can be even more addicting than cocaine.

> Sugar activates the opiate receptors in our brain and affects the reward center, which leads to compulsive behavior, despite the negative consequences like weight gain, headaches, hormone imbalances, and more...Every time we eat sweets, we are reinforcing those neuropathways, causing the brain to become increasingly hardwired to crave sugar, building up a tolerance like any other drug.[3]

Meanwhile, the American Heart Association advises to eat no more than one hundred calories' worth of added sugar per day—which is about six teaspoons.[4]

Break Sugar Addiction

One of the greatest benefits of eating God-made carbohydrate sources over man-made, processed sources is that you can break sugar addiction and terminate its effects on your health.

Have you ever been on the craving/crash cycle of sugar? You eat sugar for energy, you crash, and then your body begs for more sugar. Eating God-made carbs will help get you off this rollercoaster. Lower- and medium-glycemic carbohydrates are all God-made sources.

Sugar is highly addictive, and the more processed the sugary foods are, the more addictive they are. You're not alone if you're battling sugar addiction or cravings, but in Christ, we can overcome the tantrums of our flesh. If you refuse to feed any fleshly thing, it will get weaker. Our flesh craves whatever we give it. Picture a baby screaming for its pacifier. That is a perfect picture of our flesh!

It helps to know it won't always feel like that, and in a short amount of time, you will overcome it! Pray over your craving and replace what you typically want with a healthier behavior or option. For example, if you always crave sugar at 4:00 p.m., then get prepared with prayer and a God-made snack at 3:45 p.m.

Making over highly processed and sugary foods is easier than you think. We can make substitutions by upgrading flours, sweeteners, and trans fats for their healthier counterparts. For instance, try satisfying a sweet tooth by making a healthy apple pie with almond flour, coconut oil, and honey—or my favorite no-bake energy bites with dark chocolate chips, natural peanut butter, honey, and whey protein powder.

Here's an important key to weight loss: The more man-made, processed, high-glycemic carbs you eat, the more your body will burn sugar for energy and store fat. The more God-made, low- to medium-glycemic carbs you eat, paired with high-quality, God-made protein, the more your body will shed fat.

A Note on Fiber

When you begin to focus your carbohydrate intake on God-made foods sources like whole grains, veggies, and fruits, you will naturally increase your fiber intake and lose weight.

A study published in *Annals of Internal Medicine* suggests that something as simple as aiming to eat thirty grams of fiber each day can help you lose weight, lower your blood pressure, and improve your body's response to insulin just as effectively as a more complicated diet.[5]

Here's a real-life example of what thirty grams of fiber looks like in a whole day's worth of meals:

- Breakfast: Eggs and 1/2 cup of whole grain oats (5 grams of fiber) with 1/2 cup of blueberries (3 grams of fiber)

- Lunch: Grilled salmon with 1 cup of spinach (4 grams of fiber) and 1/2 cup chickpeas (6 grams of fiber)
- Snack: 1 small apple (4 grams of fiber) and nut butter
- Dinner: Fajita-spiced chicken with pico de gallo and 1 cup of black beans (18 grams of fiber)

Voilà! It's that simple to get in thirty grams of fiber. Did you catch that you just need to eat veggies, whole grains, or fruits with each meal?

Tips about Carbohydrates

- Avoid any programs that advocate removing all carbohydrates from your diet. This thinking is unhealthy and often leads to binge eating and giving up on your health goals. It's unbalanced and unsustainable.
- Choose a percentage of carbohydrates for your macronutrient split that matches your goals or one that naturally feels optimal for your energy needs.
- Remember that not all carbs are created equally. Choose God-made sources over man-made, processed sources; these are veggies, legumes, and whole grains that are high fiber and low in sugar. (In case you come across the term "net carbs" and you're wondering what that is, net carbs are carbs minus the fiber. Many diet plans only count the amount of net carbs in a food.)
- Fuel your temple in a way that supports your activity. For example, if you're about to work out, your body needs starchy carbohydrates—but if you're about to go to sleep, fibrous, non-starchy carbohydrates are a better option.
- Combine low- and moderate-glycemic index carbs, like fruit and starchy sources, with protein to help blunt the blood sugar response. This helps slow the rise of blood sugar and insulin,

which promotes fat storage and prevents us from using fat as energy. The goal for weight loss is to keep insulin low in the body. We do this by eating God-made carbohydrates with protein.

- To break sugar addiction, acknowledge it, surrender it, and pray over it. Replace the sugary foods you eat with lower-glycemic foods. If you do eat something with a higher glycemic index, pair it with protein to blunt the response in your blood sugar.

Chapter 14

God-Made Protein Sources

The chart on the following page is a helpful tool you can print out and keep on your refrigerator to help you make God-made choices and learn serving sizes.

Protein is the second-most prevalent substance in the human body, after water. It is made up of amino acids arranged in different combinations, is present in all cells in our bodies, and is a vital building block in the growth, maintenance, and repair of our tissues. Protein preserves energy-burning muscle tissue and raises energy expenditure in two key ways: protein digestion and metabolism. It's a win-win situation because more energy is required to digest and metabolize protein; meanwhile, protein-rich foods keep us feeling full longer than carbohydrate-dense foods, reducing our urge to consume more calories and burning off the ones we have already consumed.

Protein satisfies you more quickly, keeps you feeling full longer, reduces cravings, and helps you achieve and maintain your weight loss and muscle gaining goals.

GOD-MADE PROTEIN

God-Made Protein Sources	Serving Sizes	God-Made Plant-Based Protein Sources	Serving Sizes
Fish	3 ounces or the size of the palm of your hand	Legumes: Lentils, Peas, Chickpeas, Beans, Soybeans, and Peanuts	1/2 cup or 1 cupped handful
Seafood	3 ounces or the size of the palm of your hand	Raw and Unblanched Nuts and Seeds	1/4 cup or the size of the palm of your hand
Chicken	3 ounces or the size of the palm of your hand	Raw and Unblanched Nut and Seed Butters	2 tbsp or the size of two of your thumbs
Turkey	3 ounces or the size of the palm of your hand	Whole Grains: Quinoa, Buckwheat	1/2 cup cooked or 1 cupped handful
Red Meat	3 ounces or the size of the palm of your hand		
Eggs	2 eggs		
Beans	1/2 cup or 1 cupped handful		
Cottage Cheese	1 cup or the size of your fist		
Greek Yogurt	1 cup or the size of your fist		

Eat Proteins Close to the Way God Made Them

When you're shopping for proteins, look for antibiotic- and hormone-free, organic, grass-fed, lean cuts of meat. Choose meats that aren't fried, breaded, or packaged in heavy or sugary sauces. Read labels on dairy products like cottage cheese and yogurt, and opt for plain, unflavored varieties.

Protein is an essential component of balanced nutrition. We need to be wise when we choose our protein sources. The more we choose God-made foods, the healthier we will be.

Man-made, processed protein examples include:

- Hot dogs
- Sausage
- Bacon
- Deli meats
- Beef jerky
- Ham
- Pepperoni

Processed meats are common in our culture. Think of the typical barbeque with hot dogs, breakfasts with bacon, or the convenience of deli meats for lunch. But these meats, when preserved, form cancer-causing substances.

Eating less processed meat is easier than you think. Here are some healthy tips to get you started.

- Add grilled chicken, hard-boiled egg, beans, or tuna to your salad instead of deli meat.
- Order a grilled chicken or fish sandwich instead of a deli sandwich.
- Add vegetables or beans to your omelet instead of bacon, ham, or sausage.

Understanding Protein's Role in Your Health and Weight

I bet you've heard that you need to eat protein to lose weight, but do you know why? It's because protein reduces the hunger hormone ghrelin and boosts appetite-reducing hormones.

Other hormones are also affected by protein. Insulin (which tells the body to store fat) and glucagon (which tells the body to burn fat) are both produced in the pancreas. When one goes up, the other goes down. Obviously, we want our bodies to have more glucagon than insulin, and eating protein prompts the pancreas to do that.

The body will choose sugar over fat reserves for energy, so your goal is to keep your blood sugar low by choosing low-glycemic carbohydrates and protein to dig into your fat reserves more easily. Protein stimulates the production of glucagon and signals your body to shed excess fat.

Protein also helps you maintain and build muscle mass, feel fuller longer, and reduces cravings.

How Much Protein Should You Eat?

The answer can vary greatly depending on your goals. The Recommended Daily Allowance (RDA) for protein as determined by the Food and Nutrition Board is 0.8 grams per kilogram of body weight. This amount is the bare minimum to prevent deficiencies.

Having spent more than twenty years in the fitness industry, I know this is not enough protein to help you lose weight, gain muscle, or decrease body fat. My real-world findings are consistent with a recent study that found a protein intake of at least 1.2 to 1.6 grams per day, which is well above the current RDA, will help to promote healthy aging, decrease appetite, build muscle, and decrease body fat.[1]

Many diet programs say they have unlocked *the* secret protein macro split, but there is not a one-size-fits-all answer to what will work best for you. The answer is found in digging in with God and doing the work. Don't do what everyone else is doing; find out what works for you through prayer and application.

The best way to determine the right amount of protein for you is ask God to help you gain wisdom by walking through the How to get Fit God's Way Mini-Course then choosing amounts based on your goals: lose fat, build muscle, or maintain your physique. Determine what makes you feel best. Remember, this is a Spirit-led lifestyle of acquiring knowledge, not a flesh-driven perfection project, so practice grace, and refrain from being enslaved by numbers.

Learning the amount and sources of protein your body runs best on is an individual pursuit. Remember, through God, you have access to wisdom the world can't give you.

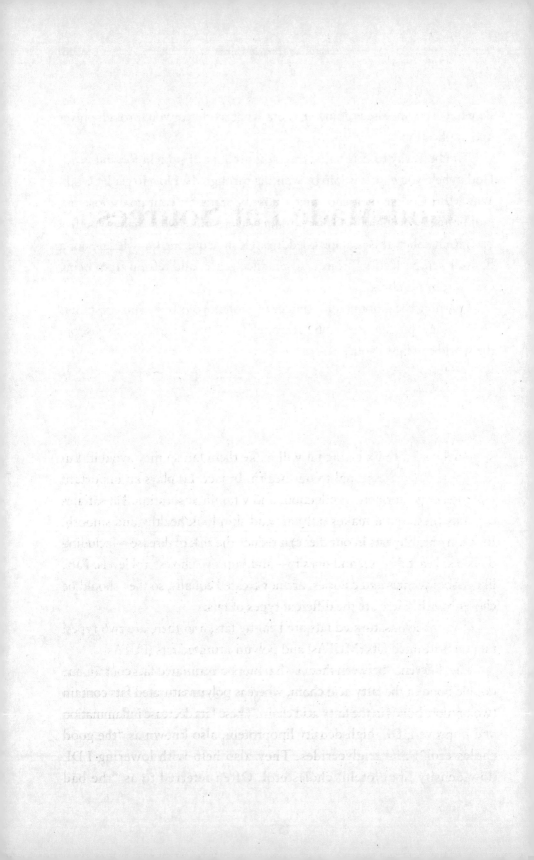

Chapter 15

God-Made Fat Sources

People often think eating fat will make them fat, so they avoid it. But some fats are essential to our health. In fact, fat plays an important role in energy, hormone production, and vitamin absorption. Fat satiates our appetites, and it makes our hair and skin look healthy and smooth. Including healthy fats in our diet can reduce the risk of disease—including diabetes, heart disease, and obesity—and improve cholesterol levels. Fats, like carbohydrates and calories, are not created equally, so they should be chosen wisely. Here are the different types of fats:

God-made unsaturated fats are healthy fats, and there are two types: monounsaturated fats (MUFAs) and polyunsaturated fats (PUFAs).

The difference between them is that monounsaturated fats contain one double bond in the fatty acid chain, whereas polyunsaturated fats contain two or more bonds in the fatty acid chain. These fats decrease inflammation and improve HDL (high-density lipoprotein, also known as "the good cholesterol") and triglycerides. They also help with lowering LDL (low-density lipoprotein) cholesterol. Often referred to as "the bad cholesterol," this type goes straight to your arteries and sticks to the walls. When this happens, it hardens the arteries, which often leads to heart attacks and strokes.

Saturated Fats Come from Both God- and Man-Made Sources

Saturated fats are known for increasing inflammation in the body, raising your risk of heart disease, and causing clogged arteries and bad cholesterol. Foods high in saturated fats are best enjoyed infrequently, so

GOD-MADE FATS

Monounsaturated and Polyunsaturated Fats

These types of fats can actually lower blood pressure, cholesterol, and the risk of heart disease.

Sources	Serving Sizes
Nuts, almonds, hazelnuts, and pecans (Monounsaturated)	1/4 cup or 1 handful
Avocados (Monounsaturated)	1/3 avocado
Olive, Peanut, Canola Oils (Monounsaturated)	1 tsp or index fingertip for cooking
Peanut and Almond Nut Butters (Monounsaturated)	2 tbsp or thumb joint to fingertip
Walnuts (Polyunsaturated Omega-3)	1/4 cup or 1 handful
Flax Seeds (Polyunsaturated Omega-3)	1 tsp or index fingertip for cooking
Fatty Fish (Polyunsaturated Omega-3)	3 ounces or the size of the palm of your hand

find healthy alternatives (a turkey burger versus a hamburger, or homemade sweet potato fries versus French fries from a drive-through).

Foods high in saturated fats include fatty meats; poultry with skin; butter, cheese, and dairy; as well as some baked goods and fried foods.

To have a healthy heart, we should enjoy saturated fats in moderation. We don't need to eat pizza or hamburgers every day, but there's nothing wrong with having them occasionally, especially if we make our own healthier versions.

Trans Fat (Man-Made, Processed Fat)

There is another kind of fat that isn't mentioned in the chart above: trans fat. This fat is made by adding hydrogen to vegetable oil to increase the shelf life of foods. But doctors consider this to be the worst fat of all. It raises both LDL (bad cholesterol) and HDL (good cholesterol). The center aisles of the grocery store are lined with products loaded with trans fat, such as

- Packaged crackers, cookies, and muffins
- Anything battered or fried
- Cakes and pies
- Margarine and shortening
- Non-dairy coffee creamers
- Prepackaged frozen meals

Tips about Fats

Our daily intake of fats should be around 20 percent to 35 percent of total calories consumed. Concentrating on monounsaturated and poly-unsaturated fats will help keep LDL cholesterol down. Monounsaturated fats include avocados, nuts, and olive oil, which all have heart-health benefits. Polyunsaturated fats include fatty fish, walnuts, and flaxseeds.

These are all high in Omega-3 fatty acids and have been shown to help fight inflammation.

Here are some examples of how to swap out unhealthy fats for healthy ones:

- Cook with olive oil instead of hydrogenated oils.
- Bake with applesauce or pumpkin puree in place of butter.
- Instead of croutons on your salad, try walnuts or almonds.
- Trade mayonnaise for Greek yogurt or avocado.
- Eat veggies with hummus instead of packaged crackers and cheese.
- Trade fried chicken for nut-crusted chicken.

Chapter 16

How to Make a God-Made Plate

As you begin the habit of intentional eating and utilizing the 7 Ps (Pause, Pray, Prepare, Portion, Practice, Plan, and Persist), the goal is to eat God-made foods in proper servings without strict dieting rules. The following tips will help you build a foundation, but remember to seek God and do what works best for you.

1. **Fill half of your plate with vegetables** (you can also add a serving of fruit once or twice a day). The more colorful your plate, the more likely you are to get the vitamins, minerals, and fiber your body needs to be healthy. Look at how purposefully God created our food:

Red Foods: Cherries, pomegranates, red peppers, tomatoes, radishes, and raspberries all contain lycopene and protect against cancer and heart disease.

Purple/Blue Foods: Eggplant, blueberries, plums, grapes, turnips, and blackberries are great for your heart and cognitive health. They fight cancer and support healthy aging.

Green Foods: Broccoli, spinach, avocado, kiwi, kale, and melons support eye health, liver function, and wound healing.

Yellow/Orange Foods: Sweet potatoes, carrots, oranges, papaya, pineapple, and butternut squash support the immune system—protecting against some cancers, aiding in heart health, and contributing to good vision and healthy skin.

White Foods: Onions, garlic, bananas, mushrooms, pears, and cauliflower are beneficial for heart health, lowering the risk of some cancers, and easing inflammation.

2. **Add a serving of protein.** God-made protein sources include not only fish, seafood, meat, poultry, and dairy, but also beans and legumes, nuts, and seeds.

3. **Choose carbs the way God made them**—whole and unrefined. These include whole grains and oats, brown or wild rice, quinoa, yams, and sweet potatoes.

4. **Add a small serving of good fats.** Try avocado slices, sauté vegetables with olive oil, or sprinkle the rest of your plate with nuts or seeds.

5. **Use spices** to mix up flavors and prevent food boredom. Choose natural, God-made ones without man-made chemicals and excessive sodium.

6. **Avoid drinking your calories.** Choose water instead of sugary drinks. Flavor with a slice of lemon, lime, apple, raspberries, cucumbers, mint, or basil.

7. **Begin to view food as a gift from God.** Look at your plate and thank Him. Choose to eat to honor Him in your body. Enjoy food from a grateful and a grace-filled heart. Skip the side dishes of guilt, perfectionism, and condemnation.

God-Made Meals, Snacks, and Desserts

Visit www.fitgodsway.com for recipes

Breakfasts

- Cherry vanilla overnight oats
- Hummus, micro greens, and diced red peppers on toast with a balsamic drizzle
- Chia seed pudding with berries
- Eggs-and-veggie omelet with sweet potato hash
- Everything bagel (avocado toast with eggs)
- Black bean, avocado, and pico de gallo burrito
- Ezekiel pita pocket with nut butter

Lunches

- Chipotle chicken burrito bowl
- Mediterranean meatballs and sweet potato fries
- Smoked salmon, avocado, and arugula salad
- Chicken, grapes, and pecan salad on romaine lettuce
- Turkey burgers with baby carrots
- Coconut curry chicken with cauliflower rice
- Fish tacos with cilantro lime cabbage

Dinners

- Balsamic salmon and roasted Brussels sprouts
- Zucchini spaghetti with ground beef, tomato sauce, garlic, and basil
- Stuffed peppers with romaine and heirloom tomato salad
- Eggplant pizza with Italian green beans
- Steak kabobs with mushrooms, onions, and peppers on coconut rice
- Turkey meatballs with spinach-and-garbanzo-bean salad
- Chicken fajitas, peppers, and onions with Ezekiel tortillas and salsa

Snacks

- Brown rice cakes with nut butter
- Greek yogurt with berries and walnuts
- Almond butter and grapes on sprouted bread
- Hummus and baby carrots
- No-bake peanut butter energy balls
- Peanut butter and apple
- Hard-boiled eggs and raw veggies

Desserts

- Dates and nut butter
- Dark chocolate with berries
- Baked apples with whole oats, pecans, and cinnamon
- Mango-lime sorbet with coconut flakes
- Fruit kabobs with pineapple, strawberries, and grapes
- Baked pears with walnuts and honey drizzle
- Pistachio no-bake bars

Tips

- We typically eat the same things, so begin upgrading your current foods by swapping man-made, processed foods with God-made, healthier versions.
- Try adding a new color to your plate each day.
- After you've learned the number of calories to eat, refrain from rigidly counting them. Avoid the diet mentality; eyeball your portions or use the hand guide method.
- Instead of stressing about finding the perfect macronutrient split, choose the highest-quality, God-made foods in proper servings.
- Don't worry about eating low-carb foods; just choose God-made carbs in proper serving sizes and fuel your body for the activity before you.

- Use smaller plates.
- When you eat out, ask the server to pack up half of your food before he brings it. Restaurants typically serve oversized portions, so we overeat without knowing it.
- Fill up on fiber. Eat those God-made veggies!
- Avoid high-calorie, low-quality, man-made foods with processed sugars, sodium, and saturated and trans fats.
- Don't drink your calories. Choose flat or sparkling water or herbal teas.
- Sit down when you eat. Set your phone aside, avoid any screens, TV, computers, etc., and focus on the meal and the friends and family with you.
- Remember, food guilt is from the enemy. When we succumb to these feelings, the stress from them could cause more weight gain than the food you enjoyed.

How Many Times a Day Should You Eat?

You may be wondering how many times to eat each day, and the answer is how your body feels best. There isn't a one-size-fits-all eating schedule, because energy requirements are different for everybody. Get to know your body and what makes you feel your best.

Here are some of the ways meals can be arranged:

- Five mini-meals
- Three smaller meals and one to two small snacks
- Three larger meals

The right answer is what works best for you and enables you to have the energy and health to feel your best each day.

Chapter 17

God-Made Snacks and Quick Meals

B ecause we're real people with real lives and we want to make this a lifestyle, there will be times when we need a quick meal, snack, or a shake. Here's a list of items to help:

1. Grass-fed whey, casein, egg, pea, or brown rice protein powders with low sugar.
2. Protein bars with limited ingredients and low sugar, like the RxBar or a Larabar.
3. Microwaveable grains and brown rice (throw in an egg, avocado, and salsa for a healthy bowl in minutes).
4. Whole-grain breads like Dave's Killer Bread or Ezekiel Bread, muffins, and pita pockets. These instantly upgrade your avocado toast or kids' nut-butter-and-honey sandwiches.
5. Chopped salad kits and pre-washed greens. Throw in a bowl with last night's protein for a meal in minutes.

6. Frozen fruits and veggies (no peeling or chopping required for your breakfast shake).
7. BPA-free canned veggies, tuna, salmon, beans, and soups.
8. Hummus (pair with carrots or your favorite veggies).
9. Nut butter packs with apple slices or celery.
10. Chopped butternut squash, spiralized zucchini, broccoli slaw, and shredded carrots all shave time off meal prep.

Flavor made easy:

- Pre-made pesto
- Salsa
- Mustard
- Hot sauce
- Fermented foods like kimchi and sauerkraut
- Herbs and spices
- Tahini
- Natural ketchup

Chapter 18

Tips for Grocery Shopping

If you're just learning how to shop for groceries and prep meals, or if you need a refresher course, these tips will help. If at any time you feel overwhelmed, remember that God has promised to be with you. Talk to Him and let Him be your strength and your confidence. It's uncomfortable to change, but remember, there are two types of pain: the temporary pain of change or the permanent pain of staying the same. Don't get stuck because you are afraid or too overwhelmed to go through this phase of learning. This adjustment period and investment in yourself is a health-and-wholeness game changer.

- Keep a grocery list on your phone and add to it as needed.
- Plan meals and snacks, and go to the store prepared with a grocery list.
- Google before you go. Look for the healthier versions of the foods you want to upgrade to save time and energy.

- Don't go grocery shopping hungry.
- Refrain from impulse buying, especially at the checkout counter.
- Read labels. If you can't pronounce it, or it has a lot of ingredients, it probably isn't healthy.
- Look for hidden sugars.
- Focus your efforts on shopping the perimeter of the store. That's where the whole foods are kept.
- Look for non-GMO, BPA-free, antibiotic- and hormone-free produce and meats.
- Buy organic when you can to avoid pesticides: potatoes, strawberries, and apples usually have the most of them.
- Buy some foods in bulk: spices, dried beans, faro, quinoa, lentils, rice, whole grains, and frozen berries.

Tips for Meal Planning

Meal prepping saves time and money and helps you eat healthier. Don't feel obligated to do it; these are just helpful tips for those who want to get started. If you think about it, you'll notice that you typically eat the same things, so making them once for the next few days is a wise use of your time.

- Choose one or two days a week to prep your meals.
- Determine how many meals you want to make.
- Start with the recipes you know, and try making them with healthier ingredients. Then build on your recipes to prevent food boredom.
- Write down the meals and the ingredients you need for them.
- Shop for groceries.
- Invest in food containers. I love glass containers with dividers and mason jars; they make food look beautiful.

Kim Dolan Leto's

GOD-MADE FOOD UPGRADES

Man-Made Food	God-Made Food Upgrade
White bread	Sprouted or whole-grain bread
Processed nut butters	Natural nut butters
Sugar and sweeteners	Maple syrup or honey
White flour	Whole-grain flour
Processed + deli meats	Fish, poultry, or beef
Highly sugary/flavored yogurt	Unsweetened Greek yogurt
Processed rice/pasta	Whole-grain/brown rice pasta
Fried/mashed potatoes	Yams, sweet potatoes
Canned vegetables	Fresh vegetables
Canned fruit	Fresh fruit
Sugary cereals	Oats, bulgur, or quinoa
Vegetable oil	Olive and avocado oils
Candy bars	Dark chocolate + berries
Regular pizza crust	Whole-grain pizza crust
Chips	Kale/apple/whole-grain chips
Trans- /Saturated-fat popcorn	Air-popped popcorn
Cookies	Baked apples with cinnamon
Candy	Dried fruit or raw nuts
Mayonnaise	Hummus or avocado
Soda (diet or regular)	Mineral water
Fruit juice	Water with fruit
Bottled artificial teas	Iced tea with lemon
Energy drinks	Green tea
Sports drinks	Ultima
Coffee with creamers	Unflavored coffee
Fried, breaded foods	Air-fried/baked/steamed foods

- Create a system. For example, bake foods like sweet potatoes and meats at the same time. While you steam veggies and rice, you can boil eggs and chop fruits and vegetables.
- Place the meals in their containers and pop them in the fridge.
- Most foods last three to four days.

Prep cooking doesn't have to be an all-or-nothing, seven-days-a-week event. Try these tips to ease into it:

- Instead of making breakfast for one morning, batch enough for the week. Overnight oats, hard-boiled eggs, egg muffins, homemade granola, yogurt and fruit parfaits, and chia pudding are just a few breakfast ideas that you can make on a Sunday and have on hand for the whole week.
- When you're making dinner, cook twice as much protein as your recipe calls for, and make one large salad. Portion the extra protein into containers for the week's lunches, and place the salad in mason jars. Simply combine the containers each day for a perfect grab-and-go lunch. (Bonus: Salads in mason jars look delicious!)
- Make a big batch of chicken burrito bowls for your lunches. These are always a favorite with my clients.
- Make lunches out of dinners with a twist. For example, if you made turkey meatballs for dinner, throw them into some salad greens and chickpeas for a quick and tasty salad. Repurposing protein for another meal always makes prep quick, easy, and healthy.
- Layer fruit into mason jars for grab-and-go snacks, and top with nuts, nut butter, or yogurt.

Make Over Your Kitchen

Prayerfully consider the foods you have in your home and the foods that you bring into it. The grocery store is your first line of defense. Set yourself and your kitchen up for success with this simple thought: You can't eat it if it isn't there. Here's how to start making over your kitchen to support your new lifestyle goals:

- Clean out your pantry of old, expired, and overly processed foods.
- Organize your kitchen to make cooking and prepping food easy. Clean out your drawers and cabinets of things you no longer use. Get drawer dividers for cooking and baking utensils. Use a revolving tray for cooking oils and spices. Place all baking items, pans, glassware, and food storage containers together in their own designated spaces.
- Keep all food other than fruit and vegetables off counters; this will eliminate impulse snacking.
- Fill a pitcher of water and add lemon or cucumber slices. Keep it in your refrigerator to encourage yourself to drink more water.
- Make a pitcher of iced green tea, flavored tea, or black tea with lemon, lime, or orange slices for another calorie-free and refreshing option.
- Keep measuring tools in the packages of foods you commonly use, like your bags of nuts, oats, and frozen fruits.
- Print out the 7 Ps and the 7 Ws, and put them on your refrigerator. You can find them at www.fitgodsway.com.
- Find a piece of home décor with an inspiring verse at a store like Hobby Lobby. Put it in your kitchen to remind yourself that you are dedicated to honoring God in your body.

Fit God's Way Power-Up Plan

Power-Up Points

- The habit of intentional eating and the 7 Ps create a healthy relationship with food.
- Fit God's Way is not a diet plan, but rather freedom from dieting.
- Surrendering our eating to God and removing food as an idol is how we repair our relationships with food.
- No diet can give us the spirit of self-control; only God can do that.
- God wants us to be wise and gain understanding. Educating ourselves about calories and serving sizes enables us to take full control of our health goals.
- Numbers are information; they are not our report card. It's important to form a healthy, grace-filled relationship with them.
- God made food to enjoy without guilt or gluttony.
- There is no one-size-fits-all approach to eating, calories, macros, or meal timing; we are all different. Invest in yourself and learn what works best for you.
- Create an environment in your home and in your life that facilitates eating God-made food and snacks.
- Dedicate your health to God.

Promises

Beloved, I pray that you may prosper in all things and be in health, just as your soul prospers. (3 John 1:2 NKJV)
Wisdom is the principal thing;

Therefore get wisdom.
And in all your getting, get understanding.
(Proverbs 4:7 NKJV)

For God gave us a spirit not of fear but of power and love and self-control. (2 Timothy 1:7 NKJV)

Prayer

Dear God,

I invite You to be Lord over my food choices. I invite You into my kitchen and to eat with me (Revelation 3:20). By the authority You've given me, I am turning away from food idolatry, body idolatry, eating disorders, body dysmorphic disorders, and any unbalanced or unhealthy eating. Let no spirit of fear find any place in my new habits. Your Word says You desire health for me (3 John 1:2), and You have given me not a spirit of fear, but of power, love, and self-control (2 Timothy 1:7). Pour Your Spirit over me as I practice self-control and choose the foods You made for my body. Let no gluttonous or guilt-induced food behaviors have any place in my life. Give me a heart for learning about servings to help me get wisdom and understanding (Proverbs 4:7). I pray that You, Lord, will be glorified in my body. In Jesus's name, amen.

Power-Up Challenge

Get Fit God's Way with the Daily 7 Ws

(Print weekly template at www.fitgodsway.com)

Word: Read your Bible and pray.

Worth: Practice placing your worth in Christ to find confidence, strength, and grace.

Whole, God-Made Food: Choose whole, God-made food over man-made, processed foods. Focus on quality ingredients versus obsessing over quantities. Pray before meals.

Water: Divide your weight in half and drink a minimum of that many ounces per day. Add seven to ten ounces of fluid every ten to twenty minutes during exercise.

Work Out: Move and strengthen your body five to six days a week. In addition, take walks outdoors to spend time in God's creation and mini-movement breaks throughout the day to increase your non-exercise activity calorie burn.

Worship: Listen to Christian music, sing, dance, and praise God.

Wake/Sleep: Establish a wake/sleep cycle and a morning/evening routine to put yourself to bed in the peace of God and wake up in His power.

HABIT 6:

Make Fitness Holy

How to Make Fitness Holy

Do you not know that you are God's temple and that God's Spirit dwells in you? If anyone destroys God's temple, God will destroy him. For God's temple is holy, and you are that temple.

1 Corinthians 3:16–17 ESV

Did you catch that? You are God's temple! That means God lives in your body. Take a moment, look in the mirror, and say aloud, "My body is the temple of God. He lives in me!" Now, doesn't that motivate you to take care of yourself?

Not too long ago, I opened my social media feed and saw a post from a Christian girl who was very sad about her placing at a recent fitness competition. She shared how she had worked out six days a week and eaten perfectly for months, but at the competition, the judges told her she wasn't lean or muscular enough.

I could feel the sadness and disappointment in her words. She said, "I thought I did everything right, I thought I looked the best I could, but I guess I'm just not good enough."

When I read her post, I hurt for her. I competed in fitness, so I knew exactly what she was going through. I sent her a message and said, "Please know this comes from a place of love and deep concern. You are so much more than body parts, a placing, or what *they* say. You are a woman of

God, and you are who He says you are. Please prayerfully consider not placing any value on someone else's opinion of you. Only God's opinion matters. Take a moment, step back from the competition, and look at the whole picture. Do you feel healthy? Do you think God wants you to feel like this? Do you think this is what being fit is supposed to feel like?"

She wrote me back and said, "I lost sight of God in this. My motivation became about all the wrong things. You have no idea how much you've helped me."

Looking back on my competitions, I can see how my motivation changed, too. It started right, but it quickly slid into frustration, desperation and, I'll admit it, number idolatry. I wanted to get healthy. I wanted to do everything I could to avoid ending up like my dad, who had a stroke, quadruple bypass surgery, and a kidney transplant before dying of a massive heart attack. I was initially scared into working out, but slowly, I saw my motivation changing. It went from working out for health to striving to make my body as lean and tiny as I could. And I felt like a failure because I couldn't maintain what I looked like at my competitions or magazine covers year-round.

> "For this is the will of God...that each one of you know how to control his own body in holiness and honor . . ."
> —1 Thessalonians 4:3–4 ESV

When Fitness Goes Here, God Is Not There!

Quite often, our motivation to work out is based on how we look and is fueled by numbers, social media likes, and attention from others. Consider the girl who shared her sadness from competing. Think of all the work she put into getting her body competition-ready, and then having people judge her for just minutes on a stage…only to go home and feel like a failure.

How Is This Healthy? How Is This Fitness?
Where Is God in Any of This?

Maybe your goal isn't to compete, but I bet you've experienced judgment from others about your body and your fitness. Maybe you've been really hard on yourself and even felt defeated. Right now, whether you are ripped and lean or overweight and out of shape, or anywhere in between, you're enough in Christ, and no one has the right to ever make you feel any less—not even your own thoughts!

Work Out Because You Love Your Body, Not Because You Hate It

Here's the problem we run into: the fitness motivation to achieve a dream body makes us think in terms of all or nothing, and it's birthed out of the wrong heart motives. It's fueled by fitness gimmicks that try to make us believe a month of working out will undo twenty years of not working out. When we don't see immediate results, we give up, and what suffers is our health. We're all in—and then we're all out. These wrong motives are why we ride the fitness rollercoaster of gaining and losing and why we feel like we are somehow less because we can't measure up to the images of fit bodies we see.

> "'For I know the thoughts that I think toward you,' says the LORD, 'thoughts of peace and not of evil, to give you a future and a hope.'"
> —Jeremiah 29:11 NKJV

The goal of this section is to make fitness a holy habit by undoing the mindsets we've adopted about fitness. I chose the word "holy" because it means *dedicated, devoted,* and *set apart.* Dedicating our workouts to God is a key difference between working out the world's way and Fit God's Way, and it speaks to our heart motives.

Have You Ever Wondered Why Your Motivation Never Lasts?

I believe there is a strong correlation between wanting to get fit and not being able to—it's having the wrong motivations. God knows our hearts, and even if we white-knuckle our way to our fitness goals and whittle ourselves down to a dream number, it never lasts. This is where we see the vanity of fitness. Did you know that "vanity" means "temporary"? Living to make your body look a certain way is just that—temporary. So often, people only look at the scale or make fitting into a certain size their obsession, but the health changes that really matter never seem to get the attention they deserve.

When you're working out but not seeing results yet, here are some of the changes that are taking place:

- Your body fat is decreasing.
- You're building muscle.
- Your cholesterol is improving.
- Your resting heart rate is getting lower.
- Your blood pressure is improving.
- You have more energy.
- You have less joint pain.
- You sleep better.
- Your skin glows.
- Your mood is better.
- You have less anxiety.
- Your stress decreases.
- You're happier.

This list shows that if we just focus on the scale or our appearance, our health suffers. Fitness is an inside-out job. The changes take place first internally, and then they're seen physically. This is why we must evaluate and often change our motives.

The Right Mindset and Motivation: Get Fit for Your Calling

The right mindset and motivation is to honor God in your body, to be the very best version of yourself so you can take care of your family and grow the Body of Christ through your God-given gifts. To make fitness a holy habit, our mindset and heart motives need to align with the Word. James sums up why fitness is such place of struggle:

You ask and do not receive, because you ask amiss, that you may spend it on your pleasures. (James 4:3 NKJV)

Could you be asking amiss? Why do you want to be fit? If you reached your fitness goals, who else's life would be changed?

Making Fitness a Holy Habit Enables You to Be Fit for Your Calling

Here are some real-life examples of what being fit for your calling looks like from women I've worked with:

- Anna takes a group fitness class three days a week and walks with her neighborhood friends two days a week. This gives her the energy and strength to volunteer at the women's homeless shelter and get down on the floor to play with her grandkids.
- Tina is a mom who lifts weights and does cardio to get the energy to run her business and take care of her family.
- Sara works out to be able to go on mission trips and work in her church's youth ministry.
- Lenora works out to stay mentally sharp and physically healthy to provide for her family.
- Erin works out to avoid diseases that run in her family, so she can fulfill the plans God has for her life.

Your calling is God's plan for your life, and being fit for it means you are taking the best care of your body—God's temple.

This level of fitness differs for everyone. For some, it may be five days a week of weight training and cardio; for others it may be cycling, hiking, or training for a marathon. But the point remains the same: being fit for your calling is motivation God can honor to help you get in the best health possible to serve others.

Five Reasons to Make Fitness a Holy Habit

- You have the best training partner in the world—Jesus.
- Your motivation is right, so He can bless your efforts.
- You're tired of fitness being all-or-nothing and quitting.
- You want to find peace with your body.
- You don't want to miss out on anything God has planned for you.

Have you heard the joke, "Paul said were supposed to buffet our bodies, not *buffet* our bodies?" Can you picture the food buffet? Not exactly what Paul had in mind when he said "buffet"; he meant to strike, to beat up. While that sounds funny, the truth is that we are supposed to be in full control of our bodies, according to 1 Corinthians 9:24–27:

> Do you not know that in a race all the runners run [their very best to win], but only one receives the prize? Run [your race] in such a way that you may seize the prize and make it yours! Now every athlete who [goes into training and] competes in the games is disciplined and exercises self-control in all things. They do it to win a crown that withers, but we [do it to receive] an imperishable [crown that cannot wither]. Therefore, I do not run without a definite goal; I do not flail around like one beating the air [just shadow boxing]. But [like a boxer] I strictly discipline my body and make it my slave, so that, after I have preached [the gospel] to others, I myself will not somehow be disqualified [as unfit for service]. (AMP)

Read that again. *I strictly discipline my body and make it my slave.* In the world we live in, I think we can all agree that most of us allow our bodies to dictate what we do way more than we should. Making fitness a holy habit is based on Paul's example; the goal is to bring our bodies under our control through spiritual training to be fit to fulfill the plans and purposes God has for our lives.

Paul Didn't Want to Be Unfit for Service

Paul, who wrote two-thirds of the New Testament, was worried about being disqualified. He wasn't worried about his eternal salvation; he knew it was a free gift from God. What he was concerned with was being disqualified for ministry. Paul wanted to be faithful and useful to God so he could accomplish what God had planned for his life. He compared the Christian life to the athletic games of that day. He disciplined his body. He ran his race with self-control. The same needs to be true of us.

Paul also mentioned being disqualified as "unfit for service." Did you know it's possible to lose your opportunity to serve God in this life because you are unfit for service? "Unfit" here relates to being intentionally unhealthy and controlled by the flesh. Our service (ministry) is our calling, the work God has placed us on Earth to do. This alone should motivate us to take care of our bodies.

Being Spiritually Fit Is How We Get Physically Fit

We must exercise ourselves toward godliness because each of us has a ministry.

> But have nothing to do with irreverent folklore and silly myths. On the other hand, discipline yourself for the purpose of godliness [keeping yourself spiritually fit]. For physical training is of some value, but godliness (spiritual training) is of value in everything and in every way, since it holds promise for the present life and for the life to come. (1 Timothy 4:7–8 AMP)

Did you know that your life is your ministry? Every day you have the ability in your sphere of influence to carry out your part of the Great Commission.

There is a direct link between our self-care and this disqualification that Paul talks about. Because we have free will, we have the ability to disqualify ourselves by living an unhealthy lifestyle.

Here are some examples:

- You can't go on a mission trip because you're not healthy enough to do so.
- You lack the confidence to sing in the church choir because you're insecure about your weight and how you look.
- You're too tired to start the business God has put on your heart because you don't take care of yourself.

God has placed us where we are and put gifts in us to glorify Him. This is our part of the Great Commission. If we don't do what Paul teaches us to do, we could miss it.

How will you answer God when He asks you, "What did you do with the talents I gave you?" Wouldn't it be an absolute shame to bury your talents under poor self-care and miss out on His plan because you were unfit for service?

> "Your talent is God's gift to you. What you do with it is your gift back to God."
> —Leo Buscaglia

And Jesus came and spoke to them, saying, "All authority has been given to Me in heaven and on earth. Go therefore and make disciples of all the nations, baptizing them in the name of the Father and of the Son and of the Holy Spirit, teaching them to observe all things that I have commanded you; and lo, I am with you always, even to the end of the age." Amen. (Matthew 28:18–20 NKJV)

Let Your Calling Fuel Your Habit of Holy Fitness

My church has a saying: "Get God, Get Real, and Get Out There!" From this saying, how would you answer these questions?

- Do you need to dedicate your fitness to God?
- Do you need to get real about working out?
- Is your health preventing you from getting out there?

Don't Miss Out on Your Calling: Finish Your Race

God has a plan for each of us, and we need our health to accomplish it. To fuel this motivation, we need to begin to focus more on what working out does for us internally than aesthetically.

Benefits of Working Out

1. Gives you the health and confidence to carry out God's plan for you.
2. Reduces your stress.
3. Increases your energy.
4. Sharpens your thinking.
5. Improves your mental and emotional health; reduces anxiety and depression.
6. Reduces your risk of heart disease, high blood pressure, diabetes, and cancers.
7. Helps you lose weight, lower body fat, and gain lean muscle mass.
8. Improves your sleep.
9. Reduces any joint pain or muscle stiffness.
10. Increases your life span.

The next time you don't see the number on the scale changing as fast as you'd like, turn your focus to all of the internal changes and benefits that are taking place. Yes, the physical changes will come, but they are the manifestation of your consistency and discipline. Don't miss your calling by choosing to be unfit for service.

For the moment all discipline seems painful rather than pleasant, but later it yields the peaceful fruit of righteousness to those who have been trained by it. (Hebrews 12:11 ESV)

Chapter 19

Work Out God's Way

Therefore we also, since we are surrounded by so great a cloud of witnesses, let us lay aside every weight, and the sin which so easily ensnares us, and let us run with endurance the race that is set before us, looking unto Jesus, the author and finisher of our faith, who for the joy that was set before Him endured the cross, despising the shame, and has sat down at the right hand of the throne of God.

Hebrews 12:1–2 NKJV

As much as I'd love to tell you that the Bible has a perfect workout plan—something like: work out for one hour a day, five days a week by taking HIIT classes on Monday, Wednesday, and Friday and weight training on Tuesdays and Thursdays—it doesn't.

But Jesus still is our example. Did you know that He and the disciples walked an average of twenty miles a day? I'm not saying we need to do that, but I am saying that our role model for living this fit life was active. He wasn't sitting around all day. He moved His body and had to be incredibly fit.

Did You Know Jesus Hiked?

Have you heard of the Jesus Trial? It's a forty-mile walk from where Jesus grew up in Nazareth to Capernaum, where His ministry was based as an adult. It takes four days to hike this trail, with each day's hike being between eight and twelve miles. Mark wasn't kidding when he said, "As Jesus walked . . ." (Mark 1:16 NIV).

When I first heard the words "Jesus Trail," I pictured a serene stroll on flat ground. I was so wrong. I love hiking, so I opened up the AllTrails app on my phone and found out this trail is hard! Picture this: In order to leave Nazareth, you have to climb straight up 405 steps. The trail has an elevation gain of 4,842 feet, and it is 40.2 miles long. And let us not forget, Jesus was wearing sandals. As a hiker, I cannot imagine how His feet felt.

Here is another example of the physical strength and cardiovascular conditioning of Jesus. Matthew 6:12 cavalierly says, "When Jesus came to the region of Caesarea Philippi . . ." It's easy to read that and not know the walk from Capernaum to Caesarea Philippi is 32.4 miles and takes ten hours and fifty-seven minutes to complete.

Don't Miss It!

Let's not allow our eyes to glaze over the names of these towns—Nazareth, Capernaum, and Caesarea Philippi—and miss the fact that Jesus walked everywhere He went. His daily life was packed with movement, and He had to have been very fit. Many of us use pedometers, like a FitBit or a Garmin, to get in a certain number of steps every day. A common goal is ten thousand steps. There are roughly two thousand steps per mile, so ten thousand steps is equivalent to five miles.

Look at how many steps Jesus and His disciples had to take to get from Capernaum to Caesarea Philippi: 32.4 miles equals 64,800 steps!

Our Bodies Were Made to Move

Although times have changed and we no longer have to walk every-where, our bodies were made to move. We need to intentionally move our bodies and exercise ourselves for His calling. Have you ever noticed that, unlike the rabbis of his time, Jesus didn't expect people to come to Him? He walked everywhere to serve others. I have to point that out, because it speaks so beautifully to His heart for us and how we need to be fit for our calling.

> As you therefore have received Christ Jesus the Lord, so walk in Him, rooted and built up in Him and established in the faith, as you have been taught, abounding in it with thanksgiving. Beware lest anyone cheat you through philosophy and empty deceit, according to the tradition of men, according to the basic principles of the world, and not according to Christ. For in Him dwells all the fullness of the Godhead bodily; and you are complete in Him, who is the head of all principality and power. (Colossians 2:6–15 NKJV)

There are so many truths in these scriptures that apply to our quest to work out God's way. Notice how it says:

Walk in Him. This means to trust Him and rely on Him, not in our ability.

Rooted and built up. This means He is our foundation, and we are built up by the Holy Spirit. We're warned not to allow people to *cheat us through philosophy or empty deceit*, which makes me think of how deceptive the fitness industry can be. And my favorite part is that we are *complete in Him.* That means, right now, regardless of where we are on our spectrum of fitness, we're enough in Him, we can have what He says we can have, and we are who He says we are.

God Is with Us in Our Workouts

One Saturday morning, I went to my favorite HIIT class, and for some reason, I was really struggling. Maybe it was because the class was really hard, or it was from a lack of sleep. Either way, I found myself staring at my shoes and wondering how I was going to make it through. As I looked down at my rose gold ASICS, I saw this:

All
Strength
In
Christ's
Sufficiency

In a crazy loud gym and a room packed with people, God showed me He was with me. He was my strength in my weakness and my friend—He is yours, too. The more we invite God into our fitness space, the more we will see Him at work and experience Him in ways that strengthen us and fuel our fitness on a completely new level.

How to Start Working Out God's Way

I appeal to you therefore, brothers, by the mercies of God, to present your bodies as a living sacrifice, holy and acceptable to God, which is your spiritual worship. (Romans 12:1 ESV)

Working out God's way requires us to shift our mindset away from self and toward Him. You may feel like your physical body and your spiritual self are completely separate, but in bringing them together, you will find deeper and lasting motivation.

Here is a list of ideas to help you work out God's way:

- Pray before your workouts.
- Ask God to help you rely on His strength, wisdom, and grace.
- Dedicate your workouts to God.

- If you feel like quitting during moves that feel hard, ask God to be your strength and to help you give it your very best effort.
- Ask the Holy Spirit to check your heart motives as you work out.
- If working out brings up things in your flesh that you're trying to overcome, remind yourself who you are in Christ. Trade: comparison for confidence, body-part idolatry for actual health benefits, pride for humility, insecurity for security, laziness for passion, and your weaknesses for His strength.
- Meditate on Scripture during workouts.
- Push yourself to be your best for Him. Don't think He doesn't care; God honors hard work when it's done for His glory.
- Focus on the internal changes, and thank God for them.
- When the physical changes come, give God the glory!
- Ask God to help you see your body as a whole work of His hands rather than body parts you dislike or want to change.
- Practice taking in deep breaths. Breathe in His presence, and then exhale your stress, doubts, and anything that's bothering you.
- Pray for the people around you at your gym or studio.
- Listen to Christian music.
- Listen to your Bible, Christian messages, or Christian podcasts.
- Put your favorite Scriptures in a note on your phone, and look at them before your workout. Pick one and try to memorize it as you train.
- Write Scriptures out and put them in your gym bag, your car, or on the walls of your home gym. Rely on them to fuel your workouts.

- When you're working out, thank God for the ability to move, bend, and stretch; how your heart beats; and how your lungs fill with air without you ever having to think about it.
- Pray after your workout. Ask God to bless your efforts.
- Build a community through Fit God's Way by sharing your go-to scriptures, favorite Christian workout songs, and the powerful difference He is making in you.
- Invite a friend to work out or walk with you. Pray together before your workouts, share scriptures, and build each other up in the Lord.
- Find a faith-based workout. You can try my *Faith Inspired Transformation Workout* on Pure Flix.

In conclusion, be strong in the Lord [draw your strength from Him and be empowered through your union with Him] and in the power of His [boundless] might. (Ephesians 6:10 AMP)

Chapter 20

Dress Yourself with Strength and Wisdom

She dresses herself with strength and makes her arms strong.

Proverbs 31:17 ESV

For the Lord gives wisdom;
From His mouth come knowledge and understanding . . .

Proverbs 2:6 NKJV

The goal of this section is to impress upon you how important you are to God. You are the manager of the temple He has given you on this earth. Your body is not your own, so it needs to be taken care of the way the owner (God) would take care of it. This means you need to take full control of your fitness so you can walk in victory. We do this by dressing ourselves with strength (physical strength) and by gaining a heart of wisdom and understanding (spiritual strength). Many of us don't know how to work out, how long to work out, or how important it is. It's not good enough to guess or to follow what someone else is doing.

Armed with Truth, Fueled by Faith

After working with women from every background, at every level, and just about every age, I've been told countless times my message sounds a lot like the fitness version of Dave Ramsey. Picture Dave Ramsey at a Total Money Makeover conference telling us to cut up our credit cards to get out of debt. I often find myself saying, "We need to get real. We need to educate ourselves. We should be the living example of what people aspire to be, because we are the body of Christ."

I find the commonalities with Ramsey interesting, because fitness is no different than finances in the aspect that just as there's no get-rich-quick scheme, there isn't a get-fit-quick scheme, either.

Think of calories as dollars. Do you see the correlation?

All the late-night, get-fit and get-rich-quick infomercials can prey on our emotions. I fully understand how tempting it is to think that there's a way to cheat the system, but do you remember what we learned in Habit 5? The Bible tells us that we reap what we sow.

If we sow reps, steps, and sweat, we reap myriad health benefits. But if we sow laziness and excuses, we reap weight gain—and in time, disease. Remember Kristi in Habit 5? I gave her the example of thinking of her weight as credit card debt she needed to pay off. Our workouts can be viewed as either a payment on the debt or an investment in our future selves. To expand upon this comparison of finances to fitness, consider paying now (workouts) instead of paying later (disease) and that neglecting our bodies is gambling with our health.

One of the 7 Ws is Working Out. In Habit 2 we set F.A.I.T.H. Goals, and in Habit 5, we calculated our BMR and TDEE. From this information, we can determine how to work out to reach our goals.

In case you're new to fitness or just getting back into it, I recommend getting a complete physical before starting any new workout regimen. If you're wondering where to start, how much to work out, and for how long, I want to familiarize you with the current Physical Activity Guidelines from the U.S. Department of Health

> "The more I made exercise about spiritual growth and discipline, the less I focused on the weight. Each lost pound was not a quest to get skinny but rather evidence of obedience to God."
>
> —Lysa Terkeurst

and Human Services. They are consistent with what I have found and are considered the flagship resource for health professionals. According to them:

> For substantial health benefits, adults should do at least 150 minutes (2 hours and 30 minutes) to 300 minutes (5 hours) a week of moderate-intensity, or 75 minutes (1 hour and 15 minutes) to 150 minutes (2 hours and 30 minutes) a week of vigorous-intensity aerobic physical activity, or an equivalent combination of moderate-intensity and vigorous-intensity aerobic activity. Preferably, aerobic activity should be spread throughout the week. Adults should also do muscle-strengthening activities of moderate or greater intensity and that involve all major muscle groups on 2 or more days a week, as these activities provide additional health benefits.[1]

Let's unpack the numbers in these guidelines:

Aerobic Activity

- 150 to 300 minutes a week of moderate activity or
- 75 to 150 minutes a week of vigorous-intensity aerobic physical activity

Strength-Training Activity

- Two or more days of weight training or
- Two or more days of bodyweight workouts (Three days is better; take one day off between sessions.)

In case you're wondering what body-weight moves are, here are some examples: Squats, lunges, pushups, step-ups, planks, tricep dips, glute bridges, and burpees. Each of these have many variations and can be done in beginner fashion all the way to an elite athletic level. To see this type of progression, imagine learning a pushup. You can start by pushing yourself away from the wall or the back of your couch. From there, progress to doing them from your knees and then from your toes. When you get really strong, try one-arm pushups from your toes. Now there's a challenge!

Let's take a look at the guidelines for aerobic physical activity. Notice there are two different intensities of aerobic exercise—moderate and vigorous—and each of them have different recommendations for time. The first is a minimum for beginners and the last is for advanced exercisers. Choose one based on your level and goals.

- **150 minutes (two hours and thirty minutes) a week of moderate-intensity aerobic activity**

Examples: walking, biking, cycling, and swimming
<u>Broken into daily requirements:</u>
25 minutes 6 days a week
30 minutes 5 days a week
37 minutes 4 days a week
50 minutes 3 days a week

For best results, I suggest adding two or more days of moderate or greater intensity strength training involving all major muscle groups. This can be done either with weights or body weight alone.

- **300 minutes (five hours) a week of moderate-intensity aerobic activity**

Examples: Walking, biking, cycling, dancing, or water aerobics

<u>Broken into daily requirements</u>:
50 minutes 6 days a week
60 minutes 5 days a week
75 minutes 4 days a week
100 minutes 3 days a week

For best results, I suggest adding two or more days of moderate or greater intensity strength training involving all major muscle groups. This can be done either with weights or body weight alone.

Or, you can opt for the shorter-duration, more vigorous, intense aerobic physical activity:

- **75 minutes a week**

Examples: running, HIIT, swimming, cycling, or jumping rope
<u>Broken into daily requirements</u>:
15 minutes 5 days a week
19 minutes 4 days a week
25 minutes 3 days a week

- **150 minutes a week of vigorous-intensity aerobic physical activity**

Examples: running, HIIT, swimming, cycling, or jumping rope
<u>Broken into daily requirements</u>:
30 minutes 5 days a week
37 minutes 4 days a week
50 minutes 3 days a week

For best results, I suggest adding two or more days of moderate or greater intensity strength training involving all major muscle groups. This can be done either with weights or bodyweight alone.

Depending upon your goal, you can decide how to structure your workouts. Here are some simple examples:

If Your Goal Is to Lose Weight

Aim for the 300 minutes of moderate-intensity aerobic activity per week or 150 minutes of vigorous-intensity aerobic activity combined with two or more strength workouts.

Here's an example of how to accomplish that:

One hour-long cardio workout or two thirty-minute cardio workouts five days a week, combined with two or more days of weight training or body weight training.

If Your Goal Is to Gain Strength

Focus on more than two strength-training workouts and choose 150 minutes of vigorous-intensity aerobic activity or 300 minutes of moderate-intensity aerobic activity based on your level.

If Your Goal Is to Maintain

Get in the required 150–300 minutes of moderate-intensity aerobic activity and two or more strength-training workouts every week.

You might be wondering how to know the difference between moderate and vigorous intensity. If you don't currently use a heart monitor or have an app on your phone that provides this information, the Mayo Clinic shares a simple way to determine your exercise intensity based on your breathing:

Moderate intensity feels somewhat hard.

- Your breathing quickens, but you're not out of breath.
- You develop a light sweat after about ten minutes of activity.
- You can carry on a conversation, but you can't sing.

Vigorous activity feels challenging.

- Your breathing is deep and rapid.
- You develop a sweat after only a few minutes of activity.
- You can't say more than a few words without pausing for breath.[2]

Working Out: One of the 7 Ws

Following the 7 Ws includes working out. Because there isn't a set workout in the Bible (or anywhere else in the world!) that I can teach you, pray for wisdom to find the workout you enjoy and the one you will stick with. Spend time with God, asking Him to share the passions He's given you, whether that's dancing, weight training, or even walking in nature. Remember that there is no one-size-fits-all workout. The best workout for you is the one you will actually do. If you need workout ideas, please visit www.fitgodsway.com.

All too often, we spend money and time on trainers and memberships only to find out what we really wanted to do was hike, cycle, or take a group fitness class at a small studio. Be true to what you hear God calling you to do, and if you're not hearing anything yet, start trying different workouts. He will help you find your exercise passion.

We've all heard we need to work out, but knowing why we should can motivate us on a much deeper level. Take a look at these benefits of aerobic and muscle-building activities, and ask God to point out the benefits that will push and inspire you toward your best health.

Benefits of Aerobic Activity

- Helps you lose weight and keep it off
- Increases your energy
- Strengthens your immune system
- Improves brain function
- Decreases your risk of Type 2 diabetes, metabolic syndrome, high blood pressure, obesity, osteoporosis, heart disease, stroke, and some cancers

- Increases circulation, which not only makes your skin glow, but carries oxygen and nutrients to your body's fifty trillion cells and removes waste
- Helps you fall asleep faster and stay asleep longer
- Effectively treats depression symptoms[3]
- Controls blood sugar
- Helps you live longer and stay active and independent as you age

Benefits of Building Muscle

- Burns more calories, even at rest
- Builds stronger bones
- Increases confidence
- Lowers body fat, makes you look leaner
- Develops better body mechanics—posture, coordination, and balance
- Makes you stronger and helps with activities of daily life—bending, lifting, stretching, pulling, and pushing
- Supports your joints, decreasing joint pain

The Number One Excuse

As you're reading over this, you might be thinking, *I don't have time to work out*. I fully understand how that feels, but the truth is we all have twenty-four hours in a day. Think about the way you spend your time. Could you create an hour in your day by limiting social media or turning off the television or streaming platform? Could you have groceries delivered or get your family to help with chores around the house? God wants us to run our day, not let the day run us. We are called to be good stewards of our bodies and our time. Ask God to reveal to you where you can steward your time and your body better.

Don't Make This Mistake

Have you heard this phrase: "Sitting is the new smoking"?

When I was writing the *Strong. Confident. His. Faith and Fitness Devotional*, I would get up really early to work out—but then I found myself sitting a *lot*! After a month of doing this, I could see and feel some unwanted changes in my body. I realized that although I had worked out, I was sitting more than usual the rest of the day. I remembered something I learned when I was studying for my fitness coaching certification. There's a fitness term called N.E.A.T., which stands for Non-Exercise Activity Thermogenesis. These are the daily activities we do, like walking the dog, cleaning the house, going to the grocery store, going outdoors, and playing with our kids. If you find yourself sitting a lot, try increasing your N.E.A.T. When you do, you will burn more calories and lose more weight. Here are some ways to increase your N.E.A.T.:

- Get a step counter.
- Play with your kids: cornhole, badminton, skating, dancing, hula hoop, or throw the football or baseball around.
- If you know you're going to be on hold or on a call, stand up and walk around.
- Take mini-movement breaks throughout your day, put on your favorite Christian song, and walk, dance, or do any movement that brings you joy.
- Don't just sit while you work. Try using a stand-up desk or a high countertop. For the periods you do sit, break it up with seated twists and arm circles, then stand up and do some squats.
- Put a foam roller by your TV and stretch while you watch.
- Take your dog for a walk.
- Stay on top of household chores.

Putting It All Together

Here's the truth: Working out may require a life change from you, but God is with you in this. Lean on Him! Make your workouts a time of worship by dedicating them to Him. This time between you and God will grow your relationship with Him and make you fit from the inside out.

Although it's tempting to wait for what feels like the right time to start working out, that time is right now. There will never be a perfect opportunity to begin working out. We often think, *I'll start when the kids grow up, when they leave the house, or when life slows down.* We wait for the right time to get fit, but the longer we wait, someday becomes later and ends up being never. Create a sense of urgency by committing your health to Him, dressing yourself with strength, and gaining a heart of wisdom. You are not alone on your Fit God's Way journey. Bring your best to Him and watch Him work!

Fit God's Way Power-Up Plan

Power-Up Points

- Making fitness holy means we dedicate our workouts to God and ask Him to bless our efforts.
- We change the motivation of our fitness from a "me" project to a "He" project.
- We work out to honor God in our bodies and to be the very best version of ourselves so we can take care of our families and grow the Body of Christ through serving with our God-given gifts.
- We work out to avoid being "unfit for service" and missing the plans God has for us.
- We take full control of our fitness by dressing ourselves with strength (physical strength) and by gaining a heart of wisdom and understanding (spiritual strength).

- We understand that the internal changes from our workouts, although unseen, are of great value and that the physical manifestations come last.

Promises

In the day when I cried out, You answered me,
And made me bold with strength in my soul.
(Psalm 138:3 NKJV)

Help me, O Lord my God!
Oh, save me according to Your mercy,
That they may know that this is Your hand—
That You, Lord, have done it! (Psalm 109:26–27 NKJV)

Many, O LORD my God, are the wonders You have done, and the plans You have for us—none can compare to You. If I proclaim and declare them, they are more than I can count. (Psalm 40:5 BSB)

Prayer

Dear God,
Give me a heart on fire to bring You glory and honor You in my body (1 Corinthians 6:20). I present my body as a living sacrifice, one You find holy and acceptable (Romans 12:1). Forgive me that in the past, my motivation to work out was separate from You. I'm beginning a new habit of dedicating my workouts to You. Your Word instructs me to dress myself with strength (Proverbs 31:17). Help me, through the power of the Holy Spirit, to turn from my excuses, laziness, and preoccupation with the

numbers and become strong from the inside out. Save me from poor health, that they may know this is Your hand—that You, Lord, have done it (Psalm 109:27). Please bless my efforts. I come to You with the right motives. My heart is sold out for You and Your plan for me. I want to be fit for my calling (Jeremiah 29:11). I pray that You would thwart Satan's plan to come against my health or tempt me to quit for any vain reasons. My strength comes from You, Lord, my rock and my redeemer (Psalm 19:14). I'm fully relying on You. In Jesus's name, amen.

Power-Up Challenge

Get Fit God's Way with the Daily 7 Ws

(Print weekly template at www.fitgodsway.com)

Word: Read your Bible and pray.

Worth: Practice placing your worth in Christ to find confidence, strength, and grace.

Whole, God-Made Food: Choose whole, God-made food over man-made, processed foods. Focus on quality ingredients versus obsessing over quantities. Pray before meals.

Water: Divide your weight in half and drink a minimum of that many ounces per day. Add seven to ten ounces of fluid every ten to twenty minutes during exercise.

Work Out: Move and strengthen your body five to six days a week. In addition, take walks outdoors to spend time in God's creation and mini-movement breaks throughout the day to increase your non-exercise activity calorie burn.

Worship: Listen to Christian music, sing, dance, and praise God.

Wake/Sleep: Establish a wake/sleep cycle and a morning/evening routine to put yourself to bed in the peace of God and wake up in His power.

HABIT 7:
Press On—Don't Quit!

How to Form the Habit of Pressing On

Brothers and sisters, I do not consider myself yet to have taken hold of it. But one thing I do: Forgetting what is behind and straining toward what is ahead, I press on toward the goal to win the prize for which God has called me heavenward in Christ Jesus.

Philippians 3:13–14 NIV

Have you ever felt like this?

- I'm so discouraged that I'm not seeing any results.
- No one notices the changes I've made, so what's the point?
- My life is so busy, I can't take care of myself.
- I'm not measuring up to my expectations.
- Why does this seem easier for everyone else?
- I'm burnt out. I went all in, and now I'm all out.
- There's got to be an easier way, this is too hard.

If you are a Jesus follower, anything you leave Him out of is going to be a place of struggle. Just this morning, I read three emails from women asking for help with their fitness.

The first one said, "Why do I keep quitting?!" The next one said, "Why can't I be consistent? I do really well for a couple weeks, but then I give up!" The third said, "Why do I always start strong, and then quit my fitness goals? How do I see it through?"

I am asked these questions daily, but today felt different. God was speaking to my heart, and He told me, "You need to tell people why they quit. It's because they have no root. Where there is no root, there is no fruit."

"[T]hey have no root in themselves . . ." (Mark 4:17 NKJV)

"You did not choose Me, but I chose you and appointed you that you should go and bear fruit, and that your fruit should remain, that whatever you ask the Father in My name He may give you." (John 15:16 ESV)

When we are rooted in Christ, His Word, and His ways, He can bless our efforts (fruit)—but when we depend on ourselves and trust our own ways, we're frustrated and unsatisfied (no root).

Meet Christine

She came to me because she couldn't stick to her goals. She would do really well for a couple weeks, but then she would quit. She asked me to help her understand why she kept quitting. I asked Christine if she had ever made God the God of her fitness goals. She laughed and said, "What do you mean? He doesn't care about the forty pounds I need to lose." As we spoke, Christine started to cry and said, "I did this to myself, I did this to my body. Why would God want to help me, and how could He help me?"

Maybe today, you feel like Christine. You've started and stopped your fitness goals more times than you can count—but you really want to see them through.

Why We Need the Godly Habit of Pressing On

Read through these and see if you can identify with this process.

1. You're excited. You tell everyone you're starting a new workout plan, diet, or challenge. You feel like this is the time you're going to do it.

2. A week or two goes by, and you see some results. People are asking you what you're doing. You feel more confident and love the attention, but you feel the adjustment. Your body is sore, you're not used to eating so clean, and your energy is low.

3. Then something throws you off: You weigh yourself, you miss a workout, you blow it one weekend, your kids get sick, or someone makes a negative comment, and you feel discouragement creep in. You start to feel like a failure, like this is impossible. You're determined to keep going, but you begin to question if what you're doing is even working or if it's worth it.

4. You start rationalizing. *Well, I don't look that bad. I'll do the next challenge—this really wasn't a good time.* These decisions are often made over a plate of nachos, in front of the TV after a long day of work, or on a morning when you'd rather clean out your closet than haul yourself to a 5:00 a.m. weigh-in and workout.

5. You start skipping your workouts and healthy meals, and days turns into weeks. You convince yourself that you'll do it next time...you know, the next challenge, or New Year's, or for your next family summer vacation.

When I share this with women I coach, they say, "It's like you're in my head, how do you know this?" I know it because I did it. I lived this way, and this cycle of quitting on myself and promising to do better next time eroded my self-confidence and my self-worth.

There's the problem: I was trying to do fitness my way by pressing on in my willpower, and it was exhausting. My fitness goals were not rooted in God, so I had no fruit. If our goals are without God, they are unsupported. He is our root. He is our firm foundation.

Break the Fitness-Failure Cycle

The truth is, this fitness journey is going to have bad days. You're going to blow it, you're going to eat things you didn't want to, you're going to skip workouts, and the scale may infuriate you—but these are just moments, and you can't allow fleshly moments to make you quit on reaching your goals.

The reason these moments shake us so badly is that we haven't connected our fitness to Christ.

To get out of the cycle, we can no longer trust in our abilities, live by our feelings, or place our confidence in ourselves. We have to recognize a bad moment is just a moment—and although we have them, they cannot have us. It's in these moments that we need to turn to God and live for Him—not the way we look.

"Leave it all in the Hands that were wounded for you."
—Elisabeth Elliot

But blessed is the one who trusts in the LORD, whose confidence is in him. They will be like a tree planted by the water that sends out its roots by the stream. It does not fear when heat comes; its leaves are always green. It has no worries in a year of drought and never fails to bear fruit. (Jeremiah 17:7–8 NIV)

How to Make Pressing On a Habit

When you make God your source, you live by the Spirit, and you have power. The Holy Spirit will speak to you, so the next time you get to a place where you're about to quit, refer to these five gut checks, and press on in Him.

1. Put God first. Have you made your body, the numbers, approval of others, or even food an idol? Confess it and put God first. "You shall have no other gods before Me." (Exodus 20:3 NKJV)

2. Say no to the unhealthy things God has highlighted in your life. Is there a food or drink that makes you lose control, or are you prideful or insecure about the way you look? "For the grace of God has appeared that offers salvation to all people. It teaches us to say no to ungodliness and worldly passions, and to live self-controlled, upright and godly lives in this present age." (Titus 2:11–12 NIV)

> "The tallest tree in the world is as good as dead without water. In the same way, the strongest Christian is nothing more than a spiritual midget without the Word of God."
> —Jim Scudder Jr.

3. Ask God to help you create healthy goals and a healthy body image. God made you. He designed you. You are one of a kind. Your identity and worth are not in fitness; they are in Christ, so ask Him what drains you of His power and steals away your progress. For example: Thinking you're a failure because of what you eat or don't eat, or how you do or don't exercise, is not of God. This is a worldly teaching that worth is found in performance, and it causes the fitness-failure cycle. "Let us examine our ways and test them and let us return to the LORD." (Lamentations 3:40 NIV)

4. Don't be double-minded. When you ask God, believe He hears you and that you have received what you asked for. We can't be double-minded. It's like straddling the fence of the spirit and the flesh; belief and unbelief. "But when you ask, you must believe and not doubt, because the one who doubts is like a wave of the sea, blown and tossed by the wind. That person should not expect to receive anything from the Lord." (James 1:6–7 NIV)

5. Choose to honor God with your free will. God will not make us make the right choices, but if we walk in the Spirit, He will help us overcome our flesh. "So I say, walk by the Spirit, and you will not gratify the desires of the flesh." (Galatians 5:16–17 NIV)

Victory Is Found in Pressing On

The song "Overcomer" by the beautifully talented Mandisa is what I'd like to use as the theme for this book. If you could see my most-played list on my phone, this song has been number one since it came out in 2013! It captures the emotions of my journey with Jesus and how He helped me lose weight, stay fit, and get free from quitting. It's the soundtrack for my Fit Sisters-in-Christ with whom I have had the privilege of working and watching God do the impossible in their fitness and wholeness.

> "The moment we come into any trial or difficulty, our first thought should be not how soon can we escape from it, or how we may lessen the pain we shall suffer from it, but how can we best glorify God in it."
>
> —Susannah Spurgeon

In Christ, we can overcome our pasts, our expectations, our daily failures, and our pride and develop the habit of pressing on, no matter what. When you're really trying to get fit, but you're not seeing any results, it can feel so hopeless. We can get down on ourselves, but if we turn to Him, He's right there to pick us up and remind us that in Him, we are overcomers. Sometimes you need to put your little holy foot down and even stomp it to claim what God has died to give you. You're going to have to fight. It's not going to be easy, but it's going to be worth it. Remember, you're an overcomer!

Meet Sue

She was addicted to sugar. Every time she ate it, she hated herself for it. It made her feel awful, but she sold out those few moments of sugary enjoyment for the headaches, the weight gain, and the energy crash, because she said it was the only time she felt happy. She asked me to pray for her and to tell her a couple things she could do to help her find joy in life again apart from her sugar fixes. Knowing she loved to dance, I told her to try a Christian Zumba class, ditch the sugar for fruit, and never eat anything sweet without pairing it with protein.

Cutting sugar from her diet was painfully hard for the first week, but then she said it got easier. It took Sue two months to break up with sugar, but replacing it with Zumba and learning to eat protein with her meals broke her sugar addiction. She told me she found a friend at Zumba, and they agreed to call each other and pray for one another if they felt like giving in to a sugary treat. I had shared the song "Overcomer" with her, so before we stopped working together, she taught me a Zumba dance she made up to go with it. She said she would put in on and dance in her kitchen and praise God for saving her from sugar.

> For whatever is born of God overcomes the world. And this is the victory that has overcome the world—our faith. Who is he who overcomes the world, but he who believes that Jesus is the Son of God? (1 John 5:4–5 NKJV)

If you need to press on today, all it takes is a moment in the presence of Jesus. Cry out to Him and tell Him about what keeps blocking your success. He's waiting to hear from you. Remember—in Him, you're an overcomer.

Chapter 21

Win the Moment: Timing, Triggers, and Temptation

Look carefully then how you walk, not as unwise but as wise, making the best use of the time, because the days are evil.

Ephesians 5:15–16 ESV

D id you know there are moments each day that could be derailing your fitness goals and preventing you from pressing on toward success?

What's Your Trigger Time?

Whether it's a nightly trip to the refrigerator, a bag of chips at 4:00 p.m., or an impulsive morning pastry when you get your coffee, we all have moments in our days that are sabotaging our goals. It makes me think about the little foxes the Song of Solomon warns us destroy the vines.

"Catch the foxes for us, the little foxes that spoil the vineyards, for our vineyards are in blossom." (Song of Solomon 2:15 ESV)

It's the little things that seem harmless, like cute little foxes—but over time, they reveal themselves as the very reason we can't reach our goals. The enemy knows exactly how to get us. He shows up to tempt us in times of weakness, and these triggers make us self-sabotage.

Think of the times throughout your day when you find yourself saying, "I need this," "I deserve this," or "I'll just have one more bite."

We tend to numb ourselves, to reward ourselves, and to use food to cope with stress, so the goal is to recognize your triggers, replace them with a healthy choice, and focus on God.

Play it out from beginning to end. How do you feel in the moments after you've eaten the sugary breakfast pastry, the whole bag of chips, the bite after bite of what numbs you? The things we often reach for to relieve stress end up worsening it. Step back and focus on the big picture to see how and when you could plan to catch yourself. I teach people to keep a note on their phone that says, "Read this when you want to give in to the things God has told you to give up." I

> "Fight every battle on your knees, and you'll win every time."
> —Charles Stanley

have my clients write out how they feel after they've indulged or record a video after they've been stress-eating and save it to watch when they're tempted to do it again. It's a powerful tool to teach yourself to stop self-destructive behavior. In these moments, the 7 Ps help us pause, pray, and center ourselves to make the choices we really want to make.

Tell God You Don't Want to Give In to Temptation Anymore

No temptation has overtaken you that is not common to man. God is faithful, and he will not let you be tempted beyond your ability, but with the temptation he will also provide the way of escape, that you may be able to endure it. (1 Corinthians 10:13 ESV)

Here is a list of common triggers:

- Running late
- Enjoying a treat, but then thinking you might as well take the whole day or weekend off from your healthy goals
- Stress, feeling overwhelmed or angry
- Wanting to reward yourself
- Not getting enough sleep
- Not planning ahead
- Skipping meals and allowing yourself to get too hungry
- Feeling alone or sad

We often don't realize that we have these health-stealing moments in our days, so take note of yours. When do you reach for something you later wish you had said no to? It's not just the food or the drinks we turn to that are the problem; it's how we beat ourselves up with guilt afterward that's so bad for our health. When I think of how my dad's life was cut short, it makes me tell myself, "I don't deserve an unhealthy treat. What I really want is to live the life Christ died to give me, all of it. I don't want to miss a thing, and especially not because of my poor food choices."

Meet Jen

She came to me because she couldn't understand why she wasn't reaching her goal. I asked her to take me through her day from beginning to end and share everything she drank, ate, and how she worked out. Jen's entire day was great, but she had a habit of taking trips to the refrigerator after everyone in her family had gone to bed. She asked, "Could the bites of peanut butter I eat at night really be derailing my progress?" I asked Jen a few more questions, and she shared that eating when everyone had gone to bed helped her relax. After I reviewed Jen's typical day, I also found she was skipping her late-afternoon snack, so this was making her hungrier at night. Her attempts to eat less were actually making her eat more, and not taking her stress to God was causing her to use food to cope. Coaching Jen to add in her late-afternoon snack and take her emotions to God helped her beat those late- night snack sessions.

What's your trigger? What's your time? Try replacing whatever you normally go to with a healthier option and prayer. God has called us to be good stewards of our bodies and our time. Knowing our triggers empowers us to wisely steward our lives.

So teach us to number our days,
That we may gain a heart of wisdom.
(Psalm 90:12 NKJV)

Chapter 22

Fasting: A Key to Pressing On

Fasting is a way of saying with our stomach and our whole body how much we need and want and trust Jesus.

John Piper

Meet Kara.

Kara asked me if she should try intermittent fasting to help her reach her fitness goals. I immediately felt my stomach sink, because my answer is not popular. I said that while it might be a diet trend for weight loss, the goal of fasting for a Christian is spiritual growth, not weight loss.

Hold on—hear me out. If you've chosen intermittent fasting and it works for you, that's great. However, I believe it should be called "intermittent eating" so we can save fasting for what it truly is—a focus on God.

Christian fasting is a spiritual discipline that helps us examine our hearts and deepen our relationship with God. We deny ourselves food and activities we enjoy to humble ourselves before God and get in tune with the Holy Spirit.

Jesus is our example for fasting: He fasted for forty days and forty nights in the wilderness. Notice that He withdrew to the wilderness to fast alone; He didn't do it to be seen. He overcame the temptation of the devil, and He showed His faith by drawing His strength from His Father.

I prayed about whether or not to add fasting to this book. It's a topic people have used to sell Christian weight-loss programs, but I think that is wrong. As followers of Jesus, we fast to know Him and His will and to grow closer to Him. Fasting takes our attention away from our flesh and puts it on the things of the Spirit, our strength.

Jesus said *"when* you fast," not *"if* you fast"—so that means it's a discipline that should be part of every Christian's life.

> "When you fast, do not look somber as the hypocrites do, for they disfigure their faces to show others they are fasting. Truly I tell you, they have received their reward in full." (Matthew 6:16 NIV)

How Fasting Affects Your Heath and Wholeness

As I worked with Kara, she shared that her husband had been unfaithful, and she couldn't bear the pain of it. Her initial call to me about weight loss was really a cry for help on a deeper level. I have found countless times that this is true. Many women ask me how to feel more confident, how to lose weight, or how to be consistent, but underneath, their question is a burden or a bondage that needs to be broken. I knew Kara needed Jesus to free her, so I shared this scripture with her about fasting:

"Direct my footsteps according to your word; let no sin have rule over me."
—Psalm 119:133 NIV

> "Is this not the fast that I have chosen:
> To loose the bonds of wickedness,
> To undo the heavy burdens,
> To let the oppressed go free,
> And that you break every yoke?" (Isaiah 58:6 NKJV)

Kara wanted to forgive her husband, but she couldn't do it in her own strength. She found herself eating for comfort and putting on weight. She was hurt that she was dealing with her pain by punishing herself. Kara felt so betrayed by her husband that she didn't want him to touch her. I shared with her that, although she asked me about fasting for weight loss, what she really needed was to fast to break the burden of unforgiveness. Kara and I agreed that she would fast one day a week. On that day, she wouldn't tell anyone about it; she would pray and meditate on scriptures to focus her whole being on God and His will for her marriage and her health. I encouraged Kara with these scriptures:

> **"At its best, Christian fasting is simply a heartfelt, body-felt exclamation point at the end of the sentence 'I love you, God. I need you more than I need food and drink, more than I need my life.'"**
> —Caitlin Riddle

> "For if you forgive other people when they sin against you, your heavenly Father will also forgive you. But if you do not forgive others their sins, your Father will not forgive your sins." (Matthew 6:14–15 NIV)

> "Come to me, all you who are weary and burdened, and I will give you rest. Take my yoke upon you and learn from me, for I am gentle and humble in heart, and you will find rest for your souls. For my yoke is easy and my burden is light." (Matthew 11:28–30 NIV)

> "But when you fast, put oil on your head and wash your face, so that it will not be obvious to others that you are fasting, but only to your Father, who is unseen; and your Father, who sees what is done in secret, will reward you." (Matthew 6:17–18 NIV)

After a couple of months of fasting, Kara was able to forgive her husband, her marriage was restored, and she was able to reach her fitness goals.

Kara's story is like many of ours. We have deep issues that we cover up, and we treat the symptoms but not the problem. I share her example because you may be sabotaging your health goals because of unresolved pain that Jesus can heal.

Fasting will deepen your relationship with God. Seek His will for how you should fast. Before you begin fasting, check with your doctor to make sure you don't have any issues that would make fasting a risk or danger to your health.

Here are some great reasons to fast:

- For a breakthrough
- To remove yokes of bondage
- For emotional, spiritual, or physical healing
- As an act of worship
- For clarity
- To seek God's will
- To show gratitude to God
- To get rid of strongholds
- For God's guidance

Ways to Fast

Giving up food is the most common way to fast, but it doesn't always have to be food that you choose to go without. What would be a sacrifice for you other than food? Here are some ideas:

- Social media
- Television
- Mainstream music

Giving up things we depend upon magnifies our focus on God.

Chapter 23

Questions and Answers

Yet in all these things we are more than conquerors through Him who loved us.

Romans 8:37 NKJV

Remember how in the very beginning of the book, I promised to be your Fit Sister-in-Christ and support you on your Fit God's Way journey? I meant it. I have a feeling you might have some questions as you start to build these seven habits into your life, so I created a space in this book where you can find answers.

Here are the most frequently asked questions:

- **How is *Fit God's Way* different than any other fitness book?**
  Fitness without God is a flesh-driven project, but in Christ, through the power of the Holy Spirit, we can live fit from a place of victory over our flesh. Trying to get fit is a battle between the flesh and the Spirit. In the flesh, it's all about what you look like, how clean you eat, and how hard you work to make yourself look good. It's fleeting, disappointing, and a form of idolatry. In the Spirit, fitness is a daily surrender of

laying down unhealthy behaviors and choosing to honor God with your body and your life to bring Him glory.

- **How often should I eat? Is it better to eat five times a day or three times a day?** There is no one answer on this, as everyone's body is different. Many fitness professionals suggest eating five small meals a day to keep your metabolism burning, your energy up, and your cravings low. However, some people prefer eating three meals a day. Try both to see which method helps you keep your energy up and your cravings down as you work toward your goals.

- **Should I fast?** Fasting is a powerful part of the Christian life. Jesus said, "*when* you fast," not "*if* you fast," so we are called to fast. Fasting is for spiritual growth—not for dieting. Please refer to Habit 7 to learn more about fasting.

- **Is working out or eating healthy more important to lose weight?** The 80/20 rule nutritionists and trainers share maintains that weight loss is 80 percent nutrition and 20 percent exercise. Weight loss comes from a caloric deficit, so if you need to burn 3,500 calories to lose a pound, think of how much easier it is to have a zero-calorie green tea than a 500-calorie mocha latte that would take an hour and a half to burn off with brisk walking. This doesn't mean we should skip our workouts, though. Working out is an integral part of weight loss and body composition changes. As we eat less, we weigh less, so our bodies adjust and burn fewer calories. Getting our workouts in helps create a caloric deficit, as well as adding and preserving muscle mass and a multitude of other important health benefits.

- **How does weight loss happen?** Weight loss occurs when you burn more calories than you eat. Wondering where it goes? We lose weight through our breath, sweat, and urine, with our breath being the main route.

- **Can I have a cheat day?** Fit God's Way is not a diet, it's a Spirit-led lifestyle. So this question is best answered by taking it to God. Prayerfully ask Him and yourself if taking an entire day off and eating everything you want is a healthy decision. While there's nothing wrong with enjoying food, we move away from godly character when we want to be gluttonous. The word "cheating" suggests that you're doing something bad when you eat, and this is not from God. God made food for us to enjoy; cheat days are a worldly dieting concept. The women I coach struggle to get back on track when they take a whole day off. I teach them to choose to enjoy one meal or treat of whatever they want, and then get back on track by making their next meal a God-made one.

- **How many days a week should I work out?** Check out Chapter 20 to learn the recommended amounts of time to help you reach your goals.

- **Do I have to lift weights?** Strengthening our bodies is vital to our bone health. It also adds skeletal muscle, which prevents injury in the activities of daily life. If weight training isn't something that interests you, try bodyweight exercises, use resistance bands, or take a TRX class.

- **Will lifting weights make me bulky?** Building muscle is hard to do, and it doesn't happen without a lot of effort and adequate protein. Looking "bulky" typically comes from a diet of man-made, processed foods. Having a consistent mix of cardio and weight training and fueling your body with God-made foods will prevent you from becoming bulky.

- **Weighing myself stresses me out. Is there another way to track my progress?** Tracking your progress is a great way to give God glory and see yourself getting healthier. The scale is one of many means to track results. Others include a measuring tape, body fat calipers, taking pictures of yourself, and trying

on a good old pair of your favorite jeans to see how they fit
over time. Whatever method you choose, celebrate what God
is doing through your health journey in Him.

- **How will I know I'm getting results?** There are many types
  of results, including emotional, mental, spiritual, and physical.
  We often quit because we only look for physical results. The
  unseen health and spiritual benefits occur before our physical
  appearance changes. Try to reframe your thinking about what
  fitness results are, because every prayer, God-made meal, and
  workout is a step closer to the healthiest and happiest version
  of you. Although the physical results will come in time, begin
  to evaluate more than what your body looks like when you're
  looking for results.

- **How do I stop my cravings?** Surrender what you crave to God.
  Never eat sugar by itself. Pair any sugary foods with protein.
  Get enough sleep. Drink more water. Keep the foods you crave
  out of your house. Don't let yourself get too hungry. Take your
  emotions and stress to God. Walk yourself through how you
  feel when you eat the things you crave and ask yourself if it's
  worth it. Replace what you crave with something healthier.
  Some studies suggest that cravings could come from vitamin
  deficiencies of magnesium, zinc, and vitamin B, so ask your
  doctor if you're deficient in any of these.

- **Do I have to give up everything I love to eat?** Eating God-made
  foods doesn't mean you have to give up everything you love.
  God wants us to enjoy food. The goal is to replace man-made,
  processed foods with healthier, God-made alternatives. For
  example, if you love to bake, use whole-grain flours, swap a
  cup of sugar for a cup of applesauce, and use 3/4 cup of
  bananas in place of 1 cup of oil. Learning simple exchanges
  creates big health benefits.

- **I have injuries; what workout can I do?** Check with your doctor to see what he or she recommends. I have coached women who chose to learn to swim because of joint pain and injuries, and others who took up cycling because of back and knee surgeries. Don't lose hope; there is a workout you can do.

- **What if I get bored from eating God-made foods?** Food boredom comes from eating the same old things, so mix it up with some new recipes or snacks, or try a healthy restaurant in your area. Spices do a lot to make over food, so if you're bored, this is a great place to start.

- **How do I stop feeling so guilty after I eat badly?** The diet mentality wants us to think that if we eat well, we are good, but if we eat badly, then we're bad. When this happens, ask God to remind you that you are not pursuing fitness in the flesh anymore, and that you have chosen fitness as a Spirit-led lifestyle. When guilt tries to consume you, let the grace of God wash over you.

- **Should I use an app to track my food?** When we first begin to understand calories and serving sizes, apps are a great tool to educate us on what and how much we're eating. Gaining a working knowledge of serving sizes is important to make Fit God's Way a lifestyle. Be cautious, though, to avoid extremes. While the information is helpful, obsessing over it can quickly become idolatry.

- **Should I time my meals?** An easy rule to follow is to fuel your body for the type of activity before you. Think about it like this: You wouldn't give a kid a bunch of sugar and send him to bed, right? So if you're going to sleep, you don't need a starchy-carb meal, either—but if you're going to work out, you do. Fuel your body with foods like oats, whole grains, and yams to support your workout and then again afterward to help your muscles repair along with some protein.

- **Why am I not losing weight?** When you first begin to work out consistently and eat healthy, the scale doesn't take into account the muscle you're building or the water your muscles are holding as they recover. Did you know you can weigh the exact same amount but look completely different based on what you're doing? This is because a pound of muscle takes up a fourth of the space of a pound of fat. Other reasons you might not be losing weight include hormonal imbalances, not being completely honest about what or how much you're eating, not giving yourself enough time to lose weight, or being inconsistent. Weight loss also stalls when we don't eat enough. It's common to think that if you don't eat, you'll lose more weight, but this actually makes your body hold onto fat. Also, our bodies adapt to our workouts and the weights we lift and the cardio we do, so we need to continually challenge ourselves with new workouts, heavier weight, more reps, or more time.

- **Does God really care about my fitness goals?** If you have accepted Jesus as your Savior, the answer is YES! God cares about every single detail of your life—even your fitness. You aren't alone in your fitness struggles and successes. You have a loving, compassionate, powerful Father to guide you. Invite Him to be the Lord of your fitness, and watch Him work.

- **I've thought about becoming a Christian; what do I need to do?** Friend, Heaven is rejoicing. Say this prayer, then find a Bible-based church in your area and tell the pastor that you are a new Christian: *Dear God, I ask You to come into my heart and be the Lord of my life. I acknowledge that I am sinful and there isn't anything I can do to earn my way to Heaven. I ask You to forgive me of my sins. I accept the overwhelming sacrifice of Your*

Son Jesus's death on the cross and His resurrection as payment for all of my sin. I trust You with everything. Thank You for coming into my heart and making me new. Thank You for hearing my prayers and loving me unconditionally—here on Earth and for eternity in Heaven. Through faith, I receive Your gift of salvation. In Jesus's name, amen.

- **I'm going through hormonal issues: perimenopause, menopause, or postmenopause. How will Fit God's Way help me?** Unbalanced hormones are a major cause of weight gain, anxiety, depression, fatigue, irritability, and many other issues. See your doctor to find out if you have any imbalances. Going through hormonal changes can be a very challenging time in a woman's life. While your emotions may want to control you, you can find peace and feel better. Following the 7 Ws will help you take the best care of yourself as your body goes through these adjustment periods. Food choices become more important than ever; sugar and processed carbs increase body fat, hot flashes, and cause myriad other unfavorable effects. Taking the best care of yourself will help hormonal issues greatly.

- **I was taught that it's vain to want to get fit or look my best. How do I get over this?** Finding your worth and identity in Christ frees you from man-made, legalistic rules. God formed you, He has a perfect plan for you, and your body is His temple, so taking the very best care of yourself and using every gift He has given you (to bring Him glory) is your assignment here on Earth.

- **I feel like it's too late and I'm too old to get fit. Is there hope for me?** God is waiting on you to bring Him glory with all He's given you. It's never too late to become the best version of yourself. Set goals, spend time with God, get in your 7 Ws, and watch Him work. You can become a new you in Him.

- **How do I get motivated?** Practice the 7 Ws every day, and notice how spending time with God in His Word and worshipping Him inspires you to honor Him in your body. Motivation comes from knowing your why. Why do you want to get fit? Here are some examples: I'm tired of missing out on God's plan for my life, I want to avoid generational diseases that run in my family, I want to be a better role model for my kids, or I want to represent God well. Stay connected with God daily, and He will help you stir yourself up through the Holy Spirit.

- **Will my arms ever tone up?** It's a myth that we can spot-reduce areas like our arms, legs, or stomach. When we lose weight, we lose it all over. However, as you follow the 7 Ws, you will notice that eating whole, God-made foods, working out, drinking more water, and sleeping better, etc., will greatly improve the way you look over time.

- **Is it okay to take the weekends off from eating God-made and working out?** Instead of taking the entire weekend off from your Fit God's Way lifestyle, plan to enjoy a date night with your husband, a treat with your kids, or brunch with a friend, but don't take the whole weekend off. Here's why: weekends are a third of the year, and taking them completely off will sabotage your fitness goals. Look at the math: 52 weekends a year x 2 days = 104 days. But if you start your weekends on Fridays, that's 52 x 3 = 156 days. With a three-day weekend, we're getting closer to half of the year. It's very hard to stop and restart a healthy lifestyle, so plan to enjoy moments, but remember the rule: no back-to-back C.R.A.P. (Cooking oils that are hydrogenated, Refined sugar, Artificial colors, Processed food).

- **I need support. Where can I find other women who are getting Fit God's Way?** Please join the private Facebook group F.I.T.

Sisters-in-Christ. Also, invite a friend and take the #FitGodsWay Challenge together.

- **I'd like to start a small Fit God's Way group. Can I do that?** Yes, and thank you for wanting to help bring women together to honor God in their bodies and make fitness a Spirit-led lifestyle. For details, visit www.fitgodsway.com.

- **What do I do if I go on vacation, get sick, or sustain an injury?** It's important to remember that Fit God's Way is a grace-filled, Spirit-led lifestyle and not a rigid diet plan. Follow the 7 Ws to the best of your ability without any pressure to be perfect. For example, if you're sick or injured, you can still get in the Word, place your Worth in Christ, drink Water, eat Whole, God-made foods, Worship God, and follow a consistent Wake/sleep routine. Focus on what you can do versus what you can't do. The same goes for when you're on vacation. Follow the 7 Ws to the best of your ability, and enjoy the gift of your trip.

- **Is there a challenge I can join?** Yes, I'm so excited that you asked. Please join the #FitGodsWay Challenge on Facebook and Instagram, and share your results to stay motivated. Don't forget to invite a friend or a group to join you so you can encourage each other and build accountability.

- **Do you have workouts available?** If you're looking for workout ideas, please visit www.fitgodsway.com. I also have beginner, intermediate, and advanced workouts you can do anywhere with modifications for all levels. You can find them at www.kimdolanleto.com; they also are streaming exclusively on Pure Flix.

- **Where can I find God-made food recipes?** God-made meals and snack ideas can be found at www.fitgodsway.com.

- **Does muscle weigh more than fat?** This is a common misconception. A pound weighs a pound, whether it's meat or a cake. However, a pound of muscle is much smaller than a pound of fat, and it burns more calories than fat. This is why you can weigh the same amount but be much smaller.

- **How do I stop allowing my body, social media, and other people's opinions make me feel like I'm not good enough?** Practice the second W, Worth. Spend time in Habit 4 learning about fit thoughts; these are thoughts that line up with the truth of who God says you are. Write down the scriptures in this section, put them on your mirror, in your phone, and in your journal. Pray them back to God and activate your faith by believing that He will free you from feelings of unworthiness.

- **Do I have to follow the 7 Ws perfectly?** Instead of thinking you have to do things perfectly, seek God for what He wants you to focus on first. Ask Him if He wants you to do all of the 7 Ws right away. Some women start with one W and add in the others over time. Other women start off trying to get in all seven each day. Practice grace by doing the best you can, and find peace in knowing that's enough.

- **How can I take the "this is so hard" out of fitness?** There will come a point when you must decide that you want the pain of change more than the pain of staying the same. God has given us free will, and the strongest and the most motivated we will ever be is when our free will is surrendered to Him.

- **Are condiments okay to add to food?** Condiments are a leading contributor to weight gain. Adding sugar, mayo, cheese, sour cream, ranch dressing, sugary ketchup, and even nuts to a meal is adding calories. Be intentional when choosing a condiment, learn the serving size, and give them a God-made ingredient upgrade.

- **Do I have to stop drinking soda?** Soda is an unhealthy weight loss and health saboteur. It spikes your blood sugar and tells your body to store fat. It also causes cravings for unhealthy food. Drinking soda daily is linked to fatty liver disease.

- **I hit a plateau; how do I break it?** Here are a few strategies: increase the time, frequency, or intensity of your workouts; get serious and be honest about what and how much you're eating; and make sure you're eating enough protein.
- **How long will it take for me to see changes?** Within six to eight weeks of consistently following the Fit God's Way 7 Habits, 7 Ws, and the 7 Ps, you will see and feel noticeable changes.
- **Can food sensitivities keep you from losing weight?** Yes! If you feel bloated, experience headaches, heartburn, nausea, or abdominal pain after you eat, you may have a food sensitivity or allergy. This can cause low-grade inflammation in your body which in turn makes it harder to lose weight. Find a doctor skilled in integrative medicine and get tested.
- **Is there a podcast I can listen to help me stay motivated?** I have a podcast called *Strong. Confident. His.* It's filled with scriptures, prayer, workout tips, recipes, real-life struggles, success stories, and more. If you're looking for daily, faith-filled fitness motivation, join me. The *Strong. Confident. His.* podcast is available on all platforms.

Fit God's Way Power-Up Plan

Power-Up Points

- We can break the cycle of starting and stopping our fitness goals with the habit of pressing on.
- We make pressing on a habit by putting God first, saying no to the unhealthy things that God has highlighted in our lives, asking God to help us have healthy goals and create a healthy body image, believing that God is working on our prayers, and by choosing to honor Him with our free will.

- There are times in our days that are derailing our fitness goals. Learning to spot these times and triggers is how we overcome them and stop them from sabotaging our health and wholeness.
- Jesus said, *"when* you fast," not *"if* you fast," so fasting is a part of the Christian life. However, fasting is not for weight loss; it is for spiritual growth.
- With any new habit, there will be many questions. Please refer to the questions and answers section to help you build your confidence that with God, all things are possible.

Promises

Rejoice in hope, be patient in tribulation, be constant in prayer. (Romans 12:12 ESV)

You keep him in perfect peace whose mind is stayed on you, because he trusts in you. (Isaiah 26:3 ESV)

But we have this treasure in jars of clay to show that this all-surpassing power is from God and not from us. We are hard pressed on every side, but not crushed; perplexed, but not in despair; persecuted, but not abandoned; struck down, but not destroyed. We always carry around in our body the death of Jesus, so that the life of Jesus may also be revealed in our body. (2 Corinthians 4:7–11 NIV)

I have fought the good fight, I have finished the race, I have kept the faith. (2 Timothy 4:7 ESV)

Prayer

Dear God,
The struggle to find the motivation to be consistent with my fitness goals has been a battle all my life. But in You, I am not a quitter. I am an overcomer (1 John 5:5). Your Word says, "forgetting what lies behind and straining toward what is ahead, I can press on toward the goal to win the prize for which you have called me in Christ Jesus" (Philippians 3:13–14). Fill me with Your presence, Father. I want to forget my past failures and recognize that I have this treasure in a jar of clay to show that this all-surpassing power is from You and not from me (2 Corinthians 4:7). Today, I'm laying down every time I've quit in the past, and I'm declaring that I am done with being a poor steward of my body. No matter what comes, I'm pressing on and promising to rejoice in hope, be patient in tribulation, and be constant in prayer (Romans 12:12). When the trials come and the enemy tests me, I will hold onto Your Word that says, "You keep him in perfect peace whose mind is stayed on you, because he trusts in you" (Isaiah 26:3). By the power of the Holy Spirit working in me, I will cross the finish line of my fitness goals and give You all the glory by saying, "I have fought the good fight, I have finished the race, I have kept the faith" (2 Timothy 4:7). Father God, it brings me to my knees to know that I did not choose You, but You chose me and appointed me to go and bear fruit, and that my fruit should remain, that whatever I ask You in the name of Jesus, You will give to me (John 15:16). I'm asking and believing and trusting in You alone to empower me to press on and have victory over my fitness, my wholeness, my calling, my everything.
In Jesus's name, amen.

Power-Up Challenge

Get Fit God's Way with the Daily 7 Ws

(Print weekly template at www.fitgodsway.com)

Word: Read your Bible and pray.

Worth: Practice placing your worth in Christ to find confidence, strength, and grace.

Whole, God-made Food: Choose whole, God-made food over man-made, processed foods. Focus on quality ingredients versus obsessing over quantities. Pray before meals.

Water: Divide your weight in half and drink a minimum of that many ounces per day. Add seven to ten ounces of fluid every ten to twenty minutes during exercise.

Workout: Move and strengthen your body five to six days a week. In addition, take walks outdoors to spend time in God's creation and mini-movement breaks throughout the day to increase your non-exercise activity calorie burn.

Worship: Listen to Christian music, sing, dance, and praise God.

Wake/Sleep: Establish a wake/sleep cycle and a morning/evening routine to put yourself to bed in the peace of God and wake up in His power.

Stop Starting Over Every Monday. Live Fit God's Way!

*I will instruct you and teach you in the way you should go; I will counsel
you with my loving eye on you.*

Psalm 32:8 NIV

Don't set this book down and think you'll come back to it another day. The time to take care of yourself is now, because the enemy wants to steal your physical, emotional, and mental health. If he can steal it, he can destroy God's plan for you and your future. The strongest you will ever be is when you are in Christ.

This promise from Jesus is our call to action:

The thief does not come except to steal, and to kill, and to destroy. I have come that they may have life, and that they may have it more abundantly. (John 10:10 NKJV)

It's time to have life more abundantly. It's time to get Fit God's Way!

Although the pages are coming to an end, your journey to get Fit God's Way is just beginning. Remember how I promised in the introduction that I would be your Fit Sister-in-Christ and give you the lasting answer for fitness? You turned the pages, buckled up your faith seatbelt, and went on the ride with me. Thank you for that. I know God can change what has kept you from your fitness goals.

Our journey through the pages uncovered seven key godly fitness habits. We began by learning how to put God first in our fitness and redefine fitness God's way. As Christ followers, Jesus is our role model for living, so we look to Him to be our guide:

- He rose early.
- He spent time with His Father.
- He prayed about everything.
- He wasn't lazy.
- He enjoyed food.
- He ate to live; He didn't live to eat.
- He walked everywhere.
- He loved people.
- He came to serve.
- He wasn't concerned with what others thought about Him.
- He lived for God and to fulfill the plan for His life.
- And He finished His race with endurance!

Our new habit of putting God first in our fitness is based on following Jesus's example and relying on the Helper, Comforter, and Counselor He gave us to live this fit life—the Holy Spirit. Making fitness a Spirit-led lifestyle instead of a flesh-driven frustration project is the turning point of greatness, and as we make this pivotal change, we discover a new hope, because God can do a "new thing" in our fitness.

Our second stop on the journey to getting fit God's way was the 7 Ws. We learned how to set F.A.I.T.H. Goals for our fitness and create a daily system of success:

- Word: Read your Bible and pray.
- Worth: Practice placing your worth in Christ to find confidence, strength, and grace.
- Whole, God-Made Food: Choose whole, God-made food over man-made, processed foods. Focus on quality ingredients versus obsessing over quantities. Pray before meals.
- Water: Divide your weight in half and drink a minimum of that many ounces per day. Add seven to ten ounces of fluid every ten to twenty minutes during exercise.
- Work Out: Move and strengthen your body five to six days a week. In addition, take walks outdoors to spend time in God's creation and mini-movement breaks throughout the day to increase your non-exercise activity calorie burn.
- Worship: Listen to Christian music, sing, dance, and praise God.
- Wake/Sleep: Establish a wake/sleep cycle and a morning/evening routine to put yourself to bed in the peace of God and wake up in His power.

We figured out that our F.A.I.T.H. Goals need a daily and weekly system that works for our lives. Without this personalized system, we lack the structure necessary to accomplish them.

The simplicity of God's ways found in the 7 Ws offers clear directions: Spend time with Him and in His Word, eat the foods He made, drink the water He gave us, find worth in Him, worship Him, invite Him to the table and to work out, and sleep in His peace and wake up in His power.

The 7 Ws are not a perfection project; they are the grace-filled roadmap for success a Fit Sister-in-Christ has been missing.

Next up was Habit 3: Activate Your Faith. We learned that faith is active. We do our part, and God does His. Just like Peter, weary after a long night of fishing, believed Jesus and let his net down again, so must we. In our world, we are inundated with "how-to" advice, but if we don't have any "want-to," nothing happens. God gives us the "want-to" when we surrender our free will to Him. Letting our nets down again and again is an act of surrendering our free will to Him. An obedient heart is what God wants from you. He doesn't expect you to be perfect. He wants you to be faithful. Faithful steps repeated can accomplish the most challenging goals. The results we long for are found in activating our faith, believing without seeing, and winning the moment in front of us.

And then my personal favorite, Habit 4: Choose Fit Thoughts. Our minds are the control tower of our lives. To win the battle in our minds, it is imperative that we think fit thoughts. Fit thoughts are godly thoughts. These thoughts line up with what God says about us. Choosing to think them guards our hearts and minds, because Jesus is the cure for what makes us insecure. The confidence our hearts long for is found when we see His perfection in our reflection.

Habit 5: Eat to Fuel Your Temple was packed with information to keep us from being deceived. The diet industry is a $72 billion a year business, so we need to be equipped with wisdom to avoid falling prey to the gimmickry of quick weight-loss fixes.

We learned one of the key takeaways of Fit God's Way: to make eating an intentional, Holy Spirit-led lifestyle instead of a diet. The 7 Ps are the tool that provide us the daily application we've been missing from our eating, and through the presence of God and the power of the indwelling Holy Spirit, we can have peace with food, joy for the journey, and self-control in the process.

Next stop was Habit 6: Make Fitness Holy. This is accomplished by dedicating our workouts to God. We do this because 1 Corinthians 6:19–20 tells us,

> Or do you not know that your body is the temple of the Holy
> Spirit who is in you, whom you have from God, and you are not
> your own? For you were bought at a price; therefore glorify God
> in your body and in your spirit, which are God's. (NKJV)

We learned to do this by dressing ourselves with strength (physical strength) and by gaining a heart of wisdom and understanding (spiritual strength). God wants us armed with truth and our workouts fueled with faith. With over twenty ways to invite God into our workouts, we are prepared to fully rely on His strength. Through the Physical Activity Guidelines, we can determine how much exercise we need for our goals. Understanding that motivation can be a daily challenge, we found a lasting solution following Paul's advice to avoid being "unfit for service" and changing our fitness inspiration from a "me" project to a "He" project.

Our last stop was Habit 7: Press On—Don't Quit! Our flesh is weak, and it will give up and quit on us, but God never will. In His strength, we can break the cycle of starting and stopping our fitness goals with the habit of pressing on. We make pressing on a habit by putting God first; saying no to the unhealthy things that He has convicted us of; asking Him to help us have healthy goals and create a healthy body image; believing that He is working on our prayers; and by choosing to honor Him daily with our free will.

Figuring out the times and triggers in our days that derail our fitness goals is how we overcome them and stop them from sabotaging our health and wholeness.

Every day you live Fit God's Way, you are successfully transforming your habits and becoming the fit and whole woman you've always wanted to be. You're going to look and feel better, but the most beautiful part of your process is the closeness and the presence of God that you will experience.

When the setbacks come, breathe easy, sweet sister. Your strength comes from the inside out. Nothing can stop you when you are powered by the Holy Spirit and your mind is set on Christ. The obstacles are bridges; they are not the end. Like a diamond is formed under pressure, so are you. Muscle grows from the weight of pressure, and good habits are born in the pressure to turn from old ways. In the moments of pressure, see that God is building something beautiful out of you. Choose Him. Choose His ways. Shift your expectations from perfection to full acceptance and assurance that you will only ever be enough because He is enough. Let that freedom wash over you like heavenly rain.

I want you to ask yourself one very important question: What will happen if you set this book down and don't take action? Remember, the enemy is after your health. Get up and fight in your Spirit! Don't let him win.

God made you, and He knows exactly what you need to succeed.

Will you believe Him and start now?

Will you put God first in your fitness?

Will you set F.A.I.T.H. goals and live by the 7 Ws?

Will you activate your faith and choose fit thoughts?

Will you eat to fuel your temple, intentionally choose God-made foods, and make fitness holy?

If you do, and you press on and don't quit, the day is coming when you will look back on the pain and frustration of wanting to get fit and find it is behind you, the bondages of dieting and perfectionism are broken, and you are free.

You have the power to reach your fitness goals. It's found in God. There's nothing you can't do in Him.

Please know that I went through this journey, so I am a sympathetic friend and sister-in-Christ who understands. I'm here for you. You are not alone in this. I have created resources, community, and a challenge to help you:

- Take the #FitGodsWay challenge by posting an image doing any one or all the 7 Ws every day with the #FitGodsWay. Show the world that you are getting Fit God's Way. Start with one or a few of the 7 Ws, and then add the others in time. (No perfection pressure here, just grace!)
- Refer to the Q&A part of this book.
- Utilize the additional resources in the appendix.
- Visit the www.fitgodsway.com website to help you take the next steps with recipes, workouts, and lifestyle tips.

- Join my Facebook group F.I.T. Sisters-in-Christ for community, support, and prayer.

Here's to You, Fit God's Way . . .

She is fit. She knows her worth. She acts in faith. She thinks godly thoughts. She fuels her body with God-made food. She makes fitness holy. She presses on through the hard times. She never gives up, because she knows she can do all things through Christ who gives her strength. SHE IS YOU!

Acknowledgments

Thank you, God, for the assignment to write this book. Father, You rescued me from the emotional pit of dieting and dissatisfaction with my body, and You set me free from perfectionism. I'll never get over the love You have for me and how You sent Your Son to die for me. My life journey with Jesus goes from glory to glory and only gets better.

Bill, you are the man God chose for me. There has never been a day in twenty-three years that I wouldn't have married you again. You have faithfully supported me through every dream! You've watched me go through my weight loss transformation, learn gymnastics in my thirties and forties, to motherhood, fitness modeling, competing, writing books, creating a workout series and a podcast, and you've sat and cried with me when we read the transformational stories from women. Throughout it all, you listen, you do the dishes, you jump in when I need you, and you have encouraged me every moment of writing this book. Thank you. I love you.

To my children, Joseph, Michael, and Giavella: I'm eternally grateful that God gave me you.

To my dad, John Dolan, who is in Heaven: without you, this book would not be. God used your strong faith and the pain of your health issues to become my purpose. Thank you for making me a hard-working fighter. I miss you so much it hurts.

To my mom, Lily Dolan: thank you for always being there to pray with me and to encourage me throughout this book. Your friendship was just what my heart needed on the good and the tough writing days.

To my very large and loving family, Crystal, Cory, Johnny, Brandy, Billy, Brynne, Tommy, Danielle, and all the kiddos: the love and support of our crazy fun family has Jesus all over it!

To my best friend, Kandace: you believe in me when no one else does, and you dream with me until it becomes a reality. Thank you for being the best, best friend.

To my Fit Sisters-in-Christ: thank you for choosing to live Fit God's Way. I have shared bits of this book with you throughout the writing process, and your prayers and feedback were the fuel my soul needed. Thank you for doing life with me. With Jesus at the center of it all, we shine through the struggles and the successes.

To Greg Johnson from Word Serve Literary Agency: Your tireless work ethic got us here. Thank you for never giving up on me.

Special appreciation to Salem Books for believing in me and this book from day one. I owe you a debt of gratitude.

Appendix

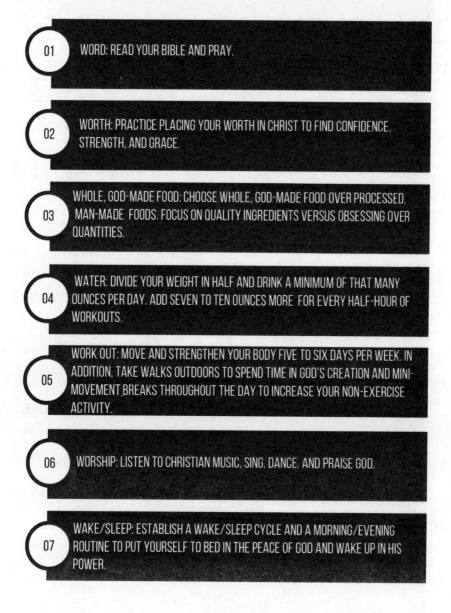

THE FIT GOD'S WAY DAILY SYSTEM : THE 7 WS

PRINT YOUR 7 WS TEMPLATE AT WWW.FITGODSWAY.COM

01 WORD: READ YOUR BIBLE AND PRAY.

02 WORTH: PRACTICE PLACING YOUR WORTH IN CHRIST TO FIND CONFIDENCE. STRENGTH, AND GRACE.

03 WHOLE, GOD-MADE FOOD: CHOOSE WHOLE, GOD-MADE FOOD OVER PROCESSED, MAN-MADE FOODS. FOCUS ON QUALITY INGREDIENTS VERSUS OBSESSING OVER QUANTITIES.

04 WATER: DIVIDE YOUR WEIGHT IN HALF AND DRINK A MINIMUM OF THAT MANY OUNCES PER DAY. ADD SEVEN TO TEN OUNCES MORE FOR EVERY HALF-HOUR OF WORKOUTS.

05 WORK OUT: MOVE AND STRENGTHEN YOUR BODY FIVE TO SIX DAYS PER WEEK. IN ADDITION, TAKE WALKS OUTDOORS TO SPEND TIME IN GOD'S CREATION AND MINI-MOVEMENT BREAKS THROUGHOUT THE DAY TO INCREASE YOUR NON-EXERCISE ACTIVITY.

06 WORSHIP: LISTEN TO CHRISTIAN MUSIC, SING, DANCE, AND PRAISE GOD.

07 WAKE/SLEEP: ESTABLISH A WAKE/SLEEP CYCLE AND A MORNING/EVENING ROUTINE TO PUT YOURSELF TO BED IN THE PEACE OF GOD AND WAKE UP IN HIS POWER.

CREATE YOUR 7 WS SYSTEM

<u>Word</u>
When will you read your Bible and pray?

_____

_____

Where will you read your Bible?

_____

_____

Will you follow a Bible plan for reading? If so, which one?

_____

_____

How will you remind yourself to pray before meals, workouts, sleep, and throughout the day?

_____

_____

<u>Worth</u>
When do you need to practice telling yourself, "I'm worthy, I'm good enough, because He is more than enough"?

_____

_____

In which places or situations in your life do you need to remind yourself that you are worthy?

_____

_____

What is standing between you and your sense of worthiness?

_____

_____

How will you remind yourself throughout the day to practice worthiness in Christ?

_____

_____

Whole, God-Made Foods

When will you plan your meals, shop for groceries, do your meal prep, and cook?

_____

_____

Where can you eat out? Which restaurants serve whole, God-made foods?

_____

_____

What processed, man-made foods can you replace with healthy, God-made foods?

_____

_____

What will you do if you overindulge? (Hint: Skip the guilt and get back on track in grace.)

_____

_____

Who will benefit from your healthier cooking?

_____

_____

How will you handle cravings, emotions, parties, and weekends?

_____

_____

Water

When will you drink water?

_____

_____

Where will you keep your water? For example, a sports bottle or glass jar?

_____

_____

What drinks need to be replaced with water?

_____

_____

How will you keep track of how much water you drink each day?

_____

_____

Work Out
What days and times will you work out?

_____

_____

Which workout will you do? Which scriptures will you take with you?

_____

_____

What will you do if you get bored?

_____

_____

What workouts can you do at home in case your kids get sick, the class gets canceled, etc.?

_____

_____

Where will you work out?

_____

_____

How long will you work out?

_____

_____

Worship
When will you worship God?

_____

_____

Where will you worship God?

_____

_____

What music and/or activity helps you worship?

_____

_____

How will you worship God more throughout your day?

_____

_____

Wake/Sleep

When will you wake up and go to sleep? Create consistent sleep and wake times.

_____

_____

Where do you need to discipline yourself to make sleep a priority? For example, what time will you turn off your phone, TV, or laptop?

_____

_____

Which scriptures can you pray back to God to help you sleep well?

_____

_____

How will you wind down? Get up? Create nightly routines and morning routines.

_____

_____

DETERMINING YOUR CALORIES WORKSHEET

It's important to remember that Fit God's Way is not a calorie-counting diet. The goal of this exercise is to help you understand calories and educate you about how many your body needs to support your goals. This is the exact exercise a trainer or nutritionist would take you through if you were paying hundreds of dollars.

You can either use an online calculator or crunch the numbers below.

Step 1. Use The Harris/Benedict Equation to determine your base metabolic rate (BMR).

BMR = (4.536 x weight) + (15.88 x height) − (5 x age) − 161
Your BMR = (4.536 x   ) + (15.88 x   ) − (5 x   ) − 161

Step 2. Choose Your Activity Level

Sedentary: I don't exercise. (Multiply BMR by 1.2)

Lightly Active: I lightly exercise 1 to 3 days per week. (Multiply BMR by 1.375)

Moderately Active: I exercise 3 to 5 days per week. (Multiply BMR by 1.55)

Very Active: I'm an athlete or I exercise 6 to 7 days per week. (Multiply BMR by 1.725)

Extra-Active: I exercise every day and have a physically demanding job. (Multiply BMR by 1.9)

Step 3. Calculate your total daily energy expenditure (TDEE). This is how many calories your body needs to maintain your current weight.

BMR x Your Activity Level = TDEE
(   ) x (   ) = (   )

Step 4. Understand caloric deficit. Let's use a TDEE of 2100 as an example.

There are 3,500 calories in a pound of fat. A simple rule of weight loss is to decrease calories by 500 per day to lose one pound per week. If we subtract 500 calories from a TDEE of 2,100, we would aim to eat 1,600 calories per day. A caloric deficit can come from a combination of food and exercise.

Step 5. Track your calories for at least a week to get a working knowledge of how many you're eating and what your portion sizes are like. Then start using the hand chart method to avoid perfectionism. This is a grace-based fitness journey.

Apps like MyFitnessPal and Cronometer are very helpful. The long-term goal is to be able to eyeball servings and avoid rigid dieting. Remember, God wants you equipped with wisdom.

CALORIE REFERENCE GUIDE

Proteins

Food Item	Quantity	Calories	Proteins (g)	Carbs (g)	Fats (g)
Beef, Ground 90% Lean	4 oz	199	22.7	0	11.3
Beef, Top Sirloin, Lean	4 oz	144	34.4	0	9.1
Beef, Top Round	4 oz	146	26.1	0	3.8
Chicken Breast Skinless	4 oz	120	26	0	1.0
Egg, Whole	1 large	70	6.3	0.4	4
Egg, White	1 large	17	3.6	0.2	0
Fish, Tuna, Chunk Light In Water	4 oz	120	26	0	1
Fish, Salmon, Atlantic	4 oz	206	28.8	0	9.2
Fish, Cod	4 oz	88	20.2	0	0.8
Fish, Tilapia	4 oz	110	23	0	2
Lobster	4 oz	102	21.3	0.6	1
Protein Powder	1 scoop	110	24	2	1
Whey	4 oz	120	23	1	2
Shrimp	4 oz	120	0	0	1
Turkey, Ground, Lean	4 oz	178	33.9	0	3.7
Turkey Breast, Skinless	4 oz	118	19	4.7	1.8

Complex Carbs (Fibrous)

Food Item	Quantity	Calories	Proteins (g)	Carbs (g)	Fats (g)
Asparagus	10 7″ spears	40	4	8	0
Broccoli	1 cup	30	2	4	0
Brussels Sprouts	1 cup	38	3	7.3	0.1
Cabbage	1 cup	21	1	5	0
Carrots	1 large	31	0.7	7.3	0.1
Cauliflower	1 cup	25	2	5	0
Celery	7″ stalk	6	0.3	1.5	0.1
Collard Greens	2 cups	22	2.1	4.3	0
Cucumber	1 small	20	2	4	0
Eggplant	1 cup	22	0.8	5	0.2
Green Beans	1 cup	33	2.6	8	0
Kale	1 cup	34	2.2	6.8	1.4
Lettuce, Romaine	3 cups	30	2	6	0
Mushrooms	1 cup	18	2	2	0.4
Onion	1/2 cup	30	0.9	6.9	0.1
Pepper, Green Red	1/2 cup	20	0.7	4.8	0.1
Salsa	4 tbsp	20	0	5	0
Spinach	3 cups	20	2	3	0
Tomato	1 medium	25	1	6	0
Zucchini	1 cup	16	1.4	3.2	0.2

Complex Carbs (Starchy)

Food Item	Quantity	Calories	Proteins (g)	Carbs (g)	Fats (g)
Black Beans	1/2 cup	100	7	20	0.5
Beans, Garbanzo	1/2 cup	110	7	19	1.5
Black-eyed Peas	1/2 cup	90	5	16	1
Bread, Whole Wheat	1 slice	100	4	20	1.5
Bread, Sprouted (Ezekiel)	1 slice	80	2	14	.05
Corn	1/2 cup	90	10	18	1
Lentils	1/4 cup	150	5	27	1
Oatmeal, Rolled Old-fashioned	1/2 cup	150	5	27	3
Oatmeal, Steel-cut	1/4 cup	150	8	27	2.5
Pasta, Whole Wheat	1 oz	105	4.5	20	1
Peas	1/2 cup	60	4	11	0
Pita, Whole Wheat	1 large	145	6	27	1.5
Potato, White	1 large	210	4.4	49	0.2
Pumpkin	1 can	175	3.5	35	0
Rice, Long-grain or Brown	1 cup	216	5	44.8	1.8
Sweet Potato	1 medium	136	2.1	31.6	0.4
Quinoa	1/4 cup	156	6	27.3	2.6
Yam	5 oz	167	2.2	39.5	0.2

Fruit

Food Item	Quantity	Calories	Proteins (g)	Carbs (g)	Fats (g)
Apple	1 medium	80	0	21	0
Applesauce, Natural	1 cup	100	0	26	0
Banana	1 medium	110	1	29	0
Blueberries	1 cup	82	1	20.4	0.6
Cantaloupe	1/2 medium	94	2.3	22.3	0.7
Grapefruit	4.7 oz	53	1.1	13.4	0.2
Grapes (seedless)	20	72	0.6	17.8	0.2
Nectarine	1 medium	67	1.3	16	0
Orange	1 medium	65	1	16.3	0.3
Peach	1 medium	59	1	15	0
Pear	1 medium	100	1	26	1
Pineapple	1 cup	82	1	22	0
Plum	1 medium	30	0	8	0
Raspberries	1 cup	60	1	15	1
Strawberries	1 cup	46	1	10.6	0
Watermelon	1 cup	50	1	11.4	0.6

Fats

Food Item	Quantity	Calories	Proteins (g)	Carbs (g)	Fats (g)
Almonds	1 oz	160	7	6	14
Avocado	1 med (3.5 oz)	161	2	8.5	14.5
Coconut (Shredded)	1/2 cup	141	1.3	6.1	13.4
Coconut Oil	1 tbsp	120	0	0	14
Fish Oil	5 soft gels	50	0	0	5
Flaxseed Oil (Supplement)	1 tbsp	130	0	0	13.3
Olives, Black Pitted/Medium	1/3 cup	50	0	2	4
Peanut Butter	1 tbsp	120	0	0	13.6
Salad Dressing (Olive Oil and Vinegar)	1 tbsp	95	4	3	8.5
Salad Dressing (Light Balsamic)	1 tbsp	75	0	0.5	8
Udo's Essential	2 tbsp	45	0	2	4
Walnuts	1/4 cup	190	7	3	18

Dairy Products

Food Item	Quantity	Calories	Proteins (g)	Carbs (g)	Fats (g)
Cheese, American Non-fat	2 slices	60	10	4	0
Cheese, Feta Low-fat	1/2 cup	120	12	0	8
Cottage Cheese 1% Low-fat	1/2 cup	100	17.5	5	1.3
Cottage Cheese Non-fat	1/2 cup	100	16.2	7.5	0
Cream Cheese Non-fat	2 tbsp	30	16	4	2
Milk, Skim	1 cup	90	8	12	0
Milk, 1% Low-fat	1 cup	100		11	2
Sour Cream Non-fat	2 tbsp	25	8 2	4	0
Yogurt, Fruit 1% Low-fat	8 oz	250	9	50	2
Yogurt, Non-fat	8 oz	100	8	17	0
Yogurt, Greek Plain	6 oz	120	18	7	0
Yogurt, Greek Vanilla	6 oz	120	16	13	0
Yogurt, Greek with Fruit	6 oz	160	19	14	3

Notes

Introduction: The Promise

1. Dolores Smyth, "What is the Biblical Significance of the Number 7?," Christianity.com, January 31, 2020, https://www.christianity.com/wiki/bible/what-is-the-biblical-significance-of-the-number-7.html.

Habit 1: Put God First in Your Fitness
Chapter 1: Redefining Fitness God's Way

1. "The $72 Billion Weight Loss & Diet Control Market in the United States...," Business Wire, February 25, 2019, https://www.businesswire.com/news/home/20190225005455/en/The-72-Billion-Weight-Loss-Diet-Control-Market-in-the-United-States-2019-2023---Why-Meal-Replacements-are-Still-Booming-but-Not-OTC-Diet-Pills---ResearchAndMarkets.com.

2. U.S. Department of Agriculture and U.S. Department of Health and Human Services, *Dietary Guidelines for Americans, 2020-2025*, 9th ed., December

2020, https://www.dietaryguidelines.gov/sites/default/files/2020-12/Dietary _Guidelines_for_Americans_2020-2025.pdf.

3. "Why People Diet, Lose Weight, and Gain It All Back," Cleveland Clinic, October 1, 2019, https://health.clevelandclinic.org/why-people-diet-lose -weight-and-gain-it-all-back.

4. SingleCare Team, "Overweight and Obesity Statistics 2022," *The Checkup*, SingleCare.com, updated February 15, 2022, https://www.singlecare.com /blog/news/obesity-statistics/.

5. "What Are Eating Disorders?," National Eating Disorders Association, 2012, https://www.nationaleatingdisorders.org/sites/default/files/ResourceHandouts/ GeneralStatistics.pdf.

6. Joseph Luciani, "Why 80 Percent of New Year's Resolutions Fail," U.S. News & World Report, December 29, 2015, https://health.usnews.com/health -news/blogs/eat-run/articles/2015-12-29/why-80-percent-of-new-years -resolutions-fail.

7. "How to Boost Your Body Confidence," Happify Daily, https://www.happify .com/hd/improve-body-image-infographic.

Chapter 2: God Can Do a New Thing in Your Fitness

1. Alisa Nicaud, "30 of God's Promises in the Bible for Uncertain Times," *Flourishing Today*, July 13, 2022, https://flourishingtoday.com/gods -promises-in-the-bible/.

Habit 2: Get Fit God's Way with the 7 Ws
Chapter 3: Set F.A.I.T.H. Goals

1. Sarah Gardner and Dave Albee, "Study Focuses on Strategies for Achieving Goals, Resolutions," *Dominican Scholar*, February 1, 2015, https://scholar .dominican.edu/news-releases/266.

Chapter 4: The 7 Ws: Your Fit God's Way System

1. Brent A. Bauer, "What Is BPA, and What Are the Concerns about BPA?," Mayo Clinic, March 8, 2022, https://www.mayoclinic.org/healthy-lifestyle /nutrition-and-healthy-eating/expert-answers/bpa/faq-20058331.

Habit 3: Activate Your Faith
Chapter 7: Tools to Help You Take Action

1. Mel Robbins, "This One Brain Hack Backed by Science Will Change Your Life. Here's How," YouTube, February 6, 2017, https://www.youtube.com /watch?v=MrZAGVq25zw&t=330s.
2. Mark Batterson, *Win the Day* (Colorado Springs: Multnomah, 2020), inside cover.
3. James Clear, *Atomic Habits* (New York: Avery, 2018), 74.

Habit 4: Choose Fit Thoughts
How to Choose Fit Thoughts

1. Relevant Staff, "How to Stop the Spiral of Toxic Thoughts," *Relevant*, August 8, 2022, https://relevantmagazine.com/life5/jennie-allen-on-how-to -stop-the-spiral-of-toxic-thoughts/.

Chapter 9: The Body Confidence Cure: See His Perfection in Your Reflection

1. CBS News, "Survey: 97 Percent of Women Have Negative Body Image," March 2, 2011, https://www.cbsnews.com/news/survey-97-percent-of -women-have-negative-body-image.

Habit 5: Eat to Fuel Your Temple
Intentionally Choosing God-Made Foods

1. Joseph Mercola, "E-Motion: Trapped Emotional Energy Is Linked to Disease," Organic Consumers Association, March 14, 2015, https://www .organicconsumers.org/news/e-motion-trapped-emotional-energy-linked -disease.
2. A. N. Memon et al., "Have Our Attempts to Curb Obesity Done More Harm than Good?," *Cureus* 12, no. 9 (September 2020): e10275, https://pubmed .ncbi.nlm.nih.gov/33042711.
3. Nicole M. Avena, Pedro Rada, and Bartley G. Hoebel, "Evidence for Sugar Addiction: Behavioral and Neurochemical Effects of Intermittent, Excessive Sugar Intake," *Neuroscience & Biobehavioral Reviews* 32, no. 1 (2008): 20–39, https://doi.org/10.1016/j.neubiorev.2007.04.019.
4. *Easton's Bible Dictionary*, 3rd ed., s.v. "glutton," by Matthew George Easton, www.biblestudytools.com/dictionary/glutton/.

Chapter 11: How to Eat God-Made Foods Mini-Course

1. M. D. Mifflin et al., "A New Predictive Equation for Resting Energy Expenditure in Healthy Individuals," *The American Journal of Clinical Nutrition* 51, no. 2 (February 1990): 241–7, https://doi.org/10.1093/ajcn/51.2.241.
2. Katie Shumake, "Nutrition and Weight: It's Personal," BeWell Stanford, January 2020, https://bewell.stanford.edu/nutrition-and-weight-its-personal.

Chapter 13: God-Made Carbohydrate Sources

1. "A Good Guide to Good Carbs: The Glycemic Index," Harvard Health Publishing, Harvard Medical School, November 16, 2021, https://www.health.harvard.edu/healthbeat/a-good-guide-to-good-carbs-the-glycemic-index.
2. "8 Principles of Low-Glycemic Eating," Harvard Health Publishing, February 15, 2014, https://www.health.harvard.edu/healthbeat/8-principles-of-low-glycemic-eating.
3. "Experts Agree: Sugar Might Be as Addictive as Cocaine," Healthline, updated April 29, 2020, https://www.healthline.com/health/food-nutrition/experts-is-sugar-addictive-drug#What-is-an-addiction?.
4. "Added Sugar Is Not So Sweet—Infographic," American Heart Association, https://www.heart.org/en/healthy-living/healthy-eating/eat-smart/sugar/added-sugar-is-not-so-sweet-infographic.
5. Nancy Ferrari, "Making One Change—Getting More Fiber—Can Help with Weight Loss," *Harvard Health Blog*, Harvard Health Publishing, February 17, 2015, https://www.health.harvard.edu/blog/making-one-change-getting-fiber-can-help-weight-loss-201502177721.

Chapter 14: God-Made Protein Sources

1. S. M. Phillips, S. Chevalier, and H. J. Leidy, "Protein 'Requirements' beyond the RDA: Implications for Optimizing Health," *Applied Physiology, Nutrition, and Metabolism* 41, no. 5 (February 9, 2016): 565–72, https://doi.org/10.1139/apnm-2015-0550.

Habit 6: Make Fitness Holy
Chapter 20: Dress Yourself with Strength and Wisdom

1. U.S. Department of Health and Human Services, *Physical Activity Guidelines for Americans*, 2nd ed. (Washington, D.C.: U.S. Department of Health and Human Services, 2018), https://health.gov/sites/default/files/2019 -09/Physical_Activity_Guidelines_2nd_edition.pdf.
2. Mayo Clinic Staff, "Exercise Intensity: How to Measure It," Mayo Health, June 17, 2021, https://www.mayoclinic.org/healthy-lifestyle/fitness/in-depth /exercise-intensity/art-20046887.
3. J. A. Blumenthal, P. J. Smith, and B. M. Hoffman, "Is Exercise a Viable Treatment for Depression?," *ACSM's Health and Fitness Journal* 16, no. 4 (July/August 2012): 14–21, https://www.ncbi.nlm.nih.gov/pmc/articles /PMC3674785.

About the Author

Kim Dolan Leto is an ESPN fitness champion and the world's leading Bible-based fitness expert. With a lifetime of Christ working in her, Kim's mission is to help women get free from the bondage of dieting and perfectionism. She knows how hard the struggle is to get fit and credits God for her weight-loss transformation and fitness success. Her book *10 Steps to Your Faith Inspired Transformation, F.I.T.* is an Amazon best-seller, and her *F.I.T. Workout* series is available on Pure Flix. Kim serves through her fitness ministry F.I.T. Sisters-in-Christ and her podcast *Strong. Confident. His.* She and her husband have three children and live in Scottsdale, Arizona.

FIT

GOD'S

WAY

by Kim Dolan Leto

Follow Kim!

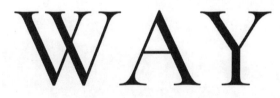

@kimdolanleto

7 HABITS

1. Put God First in Your Fitness

2. Get Fit God's Way with the 7 Ws

3. Activate Your Faith

4. Choose Fit Thoughts

5. Eat to Fuel Your Temple

6. Make Fitness Holy

7. Press On—Don't Quit!

#FitGodsWay